# A Concise Guide to Continuity of Care in Midwifery

Continuity of care in midwifery – the most traditional way of practising – has been overlooked for much of the last century but is re-emerging as an evidence-based model of care, one which is known to benefit women. This book is a vital companion to students and qualified midwives as continuity of care is integrated into midwifery education and services.

A practical, easy-to-read guide to practising caseload midwifery, this book outlines the contemporary political and professional context for midwifery care, different models of care, and the evidence and outcomes associated with continuity of carer. It discusses the real-life concerns, challenges and opportunities of working closely with women throughout their pregnancy and birth, covering key issues such as risk assessment, consent, boundaries, time management, documentation, communication, burnout and decision-making. Supporting the development of midwives from students to newly qualified professionals and beyond, it ends with a chapter containing a range of resources for reference, including helpful tools and worksheets.

Including vignettes from students, qualified midwives, and women and their partners, this book is designed for anyone new to practising midwifery continuity of care.

**Ellen Kitson-Reynolds** is a Principal Teaching Fellow and Midwifery Programme Lead at the University of Southampton, UK. She is also a Post-doctoral Clinical Academic Midwife and Professional Midwifery Advocate linked to the Princess Anne Hospital, Southampton.

**Kate Ashforth** is a clinical midwife working in a midwifery led pathway team for the University Hospitals Southampton NHS Foundation Trust.

# A Concise Guide to Continuity of Care in Midwifery

**Edited by**
**Ellen Kitson-Reynolds and Kate Ashforth**

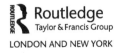

Routledge
Taylor & Francis Group

LONDON AND NEW YORK

First published 2022
by Routledge
2 Park Square, Milton Park, Abingdon, Oxon OX14 4RN

and by Routledge
52 Vanderbilt Avenue, New York, NY 10017

*Routledge is an imprint of the Taylor & Francis Group, an informa business*

*British Library Cataloguing in Publication Data*
A catalogue record for this book is available from the British Library

*Library of Congress Cataloging-in-Publication Data*
Names: Kitson-Reynolds, Ellen, editor. | Ashforth, Kate, editor.
Title: A concise guide to continuity of care in midwifery / edited by
    Ellen Kitson-Reynolds and Kate Ashforth.
Description: Milton Park, Abingdon, Oxon ; New York, NY : Routledge, 2021. |
    Includes bibliographical references and index. | Summary: "Continuity of care in
    midwifery - the most traditional way of practising - has been overlooked for much of
    the last century but is re-emerging as an evidence-based model of care, one which is
    known to benefit women. This book is a vital companion to students and qualified
    midwives as continuity of care is integrated into midwifery education and services.
    Including vignettes from students, qualified midwives, and women and their partners,
    this book is designed for anyone new to practising midwifery continuity of care"–
    Provided by publisher.
Identifiers: LCCN 2021006000 (print) | LCCN 2021006001 (ebook) | ISBN
    9780367508463 (hardback) | ISBN 9780367508470 (paperback) | ISBN
    9781003051527 (ebook)
Subjects: LCSH: Midwifery.
Classification: LCC RG950 .C63 2021  (print) | LCC RG950  (ebook) | DDC
    618.2–dc23
LC record available at https://lccn.loc.gov/2021006000
LC ebook record available at https://lccn.loc.gov/2021006001

ISBN: 978-0-367-50846-3 (hbk)
ISBN: 978-0-367-50847-0 (pbk)
ISBN: 978-1-003-05152-7 (ebk)

DOI: 10.4324/9781003051527

Typeset in Times New Roman
by Taylor & Francis Books

Dedicated to Simon, "a day without you is not a day to be had"

# Contents

# Figures

# Tables

# Boxes

# Contributors

**Ellen Kitson-Reynolds** is a Principal Teaching Fellow, Midwifery Programmes Lead and Manager, Lead Midwife for Education at the University of Southampton. She is also a Professional Midwifery Advocate linked to the University Hospital Southampton NHS Foundation Trust. Her interests link to transition, bladder management and autonomous practice.

**Kate Ashforth** is a clinical midwife working in a midwifery led pathway team at the University Hospital Southampton NHS Foundation Trust.

**Emer Kelly** is a Senior Teaching Fellow at the University of Southampton. Emer's background is in Nursing (Women's health promotion) and high-risk midwifery care in her role as a Clinical Midwifery Manager. Emer is passionate about women's psychological wellbeing during pregnancy, intrapartum and postpartum period. She module leads Obstetric Emergencies and Newborn and Infant Physical Examination. Working clinically she ensures her updated practice is reflected in her teaching to equip students with the knowledge and confidence to support women and their families throughout their child-birth experience. Emer is currently conducting research into the impact of feedback on student life experience.

**Marie Naish** is a Senior Teaching Fellow at the University of Southampton. Her clinical background includes caseload held midwifery practice, providing antenatal, intrapartum and postnatal care to women and families aged 18 and under. Marie has a passion for reducing social and health inequalities. She leads a module exploring maternity care and health promotion for vulnerable families during pregnancy and beyond. Marie supports students undertaking their caseload held experience in clinical practice. Marie is currently undertaking her doctoral study exploring the experiences of women, birth partners and midwives of a dedicated, 24-hour, telephone support line for labour.

**Maggie O'Brien** has held senior midwifery leadership positions both in the UK and NZ, including the Director of Midwifery for Imperial College Healthcare NHS Trust and more recently for Auckland District Health Board. She has extensive knowledge of midwifery models of care (including continuity of care) both countries. Maggie was elected President of the Royal College of Midwives from 2004 until 2008 and received an Honorary Fellowship from them in 2009. She is currently a Senior Teaching Fellow at the University of Southampton and believes strongly in the importance of developing compassionate cultures for both women and midwives.

**Lesley Turner** is a Senior Teaching Fellow at the University of Southampton and will be supporting students as they undertake caseload midwifery. She has previously undertaken systematic literature reviews and has a keen interest in safe staffing in midwifery. She has previously taught public health modules focusing on inequalities in health outcomes. Lesley is a promoter of caseload midwifery, due to the potential for improved physical and mental health outcomes and to improve life-chances in vulnerable groups.

# Acknowledgements

The authors of this book wish to acknowledge and thank all student midwives, women, qualified midwives, midwife teachers, service providers and researchers for their continued devotion to enhancing safe, high quality care for women and their families around the globe. Continuity of carer takes this to the next level. Thank you all.

# List of abbreviations

| | |
|---|---|
| AEI | Approved Education Institution |
| AIMS | Association for Improvements in Maternity Services |
| AMU | Alongside Midwifery-Led Unit |
| BAME | Black, Asian, Minority Ethnic |
| CLIP | Collaborative Learning in Practice |
| COSMOS | COmparing Standard Maternity care with One-to-one midwifery Support |
| DH | Department of Health |
| EXON | Examination of the Newborn |
| FMU | Freestanding Midwifery-Led Unit |
| ICM | International Confederation of Midwives |
| LMC | Lead Maternity Carers |
| MERAS | Midwifery Employee Representative and Advisory Service |
| MORA | Midwifery Ongoing Record of Achievement |
| NCT | National Childbirth Trust |
| NHS | National Health Service |
| NHSE | National Health Service England |
| NICE | National Institute for Health and Care Excellence |
| NIPE | Newborn Infant Physical Examination |
| NMC | Nursing and Midwifery Council |
| NZ | New Zealand |
| NZCOM | New Zealand College of Midwives |
| PMA | Professional Midwifery Advocate |
| POPPIE | Pilot study Of midwifery Practice in Preterm birth Including women's Experiences |
| RCM | Royal College of Midwives |
| RCS | Restorative Clinical Supervision |
| RCT | Randomised Controlled Trial |
| SSSA | Standards for Student Supervision and Assessment |
| TUC | Trade Union Congress |
| UK | United Kingdom |
| VBE | Values Based Enquiry |
| WHO | World Health Organisation |

# 1 Introduction

*Ellen Kitson-Reynolds*

## Introduction

Midwifery, as a global profession, provides care for women throughout the childbirth continuum, newborn infants, partners, and families in all care settings (World Health Organisation (WHO), 2019). Midwives across the globe have the ability to enhance quality care, reducing maternal and newborn mortality and morbidity through engaging with quality, lifelong education (Nursing and Midwifery Council (NMC), 2019). Through an initial period of high-level education, as a student midwife, you have agreed to embark on a lifelong journey of self and reflective learning and discovery. As you navigate your way through challenging, emotional, personal yet rewarding circumstances, your self-less giving to your profession and more importantly women locally, nationally, and internationally, will undoubtedly result in 'better' outcomes and greater satisfaction for all involved in this partnership. The implementation of the Better Births (NHS England, 2016b) recommendations is impacting all maternity services and midwives' working patterns. You are at the centre of continuity of carer policy implementation. Ultimately, you will have developed resilience skills required to enhance overall public health and wellbeing, thus supporting women and their families through their next generations to come. The NMC (2019) 'Standards for Pre-Registration Midwifery Programmes' and International Confederation of Midwives (ICM) (2017) ensure that:

> The midwife is recognised as a responsible and accountable professional who works in partnership with women to give the necessary support, care and advice during pregnancy, labour and the postpartum period, to conduct births on the midwife's own responsibility and to provide care for the newborn and the infant. This care includes preventative measures, the promotion of normal birth, the detection of complications in mother and child, the accessing of medical care or other appropriate assistance and the carrying out of emergency measures.
>
> (ICM, 2017)

The book is for anyone who is interested in midwifery practice and it is underpinned by a set of beliefs and values that espouse a 'humanised' holistic woman centred approach to care, provided by competent and knowledgeable practitioners with kindness, compassion, trustworthiness, respect and a nurturing manner. Throughout this book, the use of the term 'woman/women' refers to all those individuals who are pregnant and/or birthing. It is the intention of the authors throughout to recognise the

DOI: 10.4324/9781003051527-1

diversity of people who may or may not identify as women. This is consistent with the principles of the 6 Cs (Cummings and Bennett, 2012), Better Births (NHS England, 2016b), the United Kingdom's (UK) National Health Service (NHS) five-year plan (2019), the NHS Constitution (Department of Health, 2015), The Lancet series for midwifery (Renfrew et al., 2014) and the ICM (2017; 2010) definition of a midwife. This book has adopted a values-based approach from recruitment through to lifelong learning. It recognises the need for midwives to have a clear vision of their own potential to promote excellence, embrace a greater public health role and to meet the challenges of reducing global to local inequalities and improving maternal and family health and well-being thus incorporating the evidence-informed framework for maternal and newborn care (Renfrew et al., 2014). For those of you completing the activities throughout this book, you will be able to demonstrate the strength, flexibility and resourcefulness required to work in stressful, difficult yet rewarding situations (NMC, 2019a). You will have the potential to become future leaders within the midwifery profession with capabilities to respond flexibly and effectively, to the changes and technological advances in the health care environment.

Your local, national, and international midwifery colleagues are committed to the provision of high-quality education that is responsive to the changing state and knowledge in health and midwifery provision, and to meet client needs and expectations (WHO, 2019; The Lancet Series, 2014; NHS England, 2016b) to support the future workforce. In essence, midwives work together as one big 'family' to support the future of the profession and ultimately the safe delivery of care excellence for all women and their families. As a midwife, you have the opportunity, and indeed are expected, to develop an evidence informed approach to care provision (NMC, 2015; WHO, 2019; Ciliska et al., 2010)

---

**Box 1.1  Activity 1.1**

By the end of this introductory chapter, you will have started to devise your personal philosophy of care. As you read each section make a list of the things that hold a strong truth to your personal values and beliefs, and why you have decided to become a midwife.

---

For many women, midwives are the first or main health care professional that they and their family will have encountered. Within many communities, and through changing levels of austerity, many families live with several generations in one residence (Tapper, 2019; Office for National Statistics, 2019). It is likely that midwives will be the main healthcare professional providing health promotion advice and education for the whole family. Midwives are likely, therefore, to be the person who risk assesses the family environment and identifies where assistance may be required. An example of this would be where an elderly family member resides with younger family and may be subtly developing dementia or Alzheimer's, but the family may not have realised this or, as the level of care increases, they are not aware of the social support that may be available to support them in continuing to provide safe care at home. This will impact on the level of mental well-being for the whole family which may then impact on the safeguarding of the unborn baby. Whilst this appears dramatic as an example, it remains a reality for many families. It is essential therefore, that midwives have knowledge on wider health and social care issues to signpost families to the multi-disciplinary team, thus role modelling positive health care support systems for the wider family. How does this fit with case-loading or continuity of carer models I hear you ask? Well, families who build a relationship with a known and consistent carer are more likely to trust and disclose (Huber and Sandall, 2006). The midwife is more likely to elicit information from other forms of communication, not just verbal, through serial contacts. The power of observation cannot be underestimated for sub-conscious decision-making processes in these circumstances (Kitson-Reynolds, 2010). This will be considered further throughout the chapters.

## Who is this resource for?

This resource has been crafted to support the development of your midwifery professional prowess and provide you with the detailed knowledge and skills necessary to equip you for a career in Midwifery (NHS England, 2016b; NHS five-year plan, 2019; The Lancet Series, 2014; WHO, 2019). It is anticipated that the readership is predominantly, although not exclusively, UK-based and thus the book aims to develop your competence in applying professional skills to the autonomous practice of typical midwifery in accordance with the 'The Code: Standards of conduct, performance and ethics for nurses and midwives' (NMC 2015 updated 2018).

The compilation has been written as a resource to support you from the first day of the first year of your pre-registration midwifery programme through to your pre-ceptorship period and beyond as a qualified midwife. Whilst the initial intention is to achieve a continuity of carer skills base, the content of the book aims to equip you with skills for contemporary midwifery practice regardless, hence you may recommend this text to your qualified clinical colleagues as well as your peers.

Although the focus is primarily on student midwives through their pre-registration education, others such as midwife educators, academic assessors, qualified and practising midwives, practice educators, Local Maternity Systems and continuity of carer implementation teams, front line health care professionals and Doulas may also find usefulness with the content.

## How to use this resource

The book has been constructed as a companion for you throughout your course as a student midwife taking you into your preceptorship period as a newly qualified midwife and your future practice as a practice supervisor/assessor supporting the next generation of midwives and workforce. Your Approved Education Institution (AEI) will be invested in a research and evidence-based approach to its education delivery that cares about the real world and how research changes the world we inhabit. Your learning will follow an inclusive evidence-based approach and you will develop the research knowledge and skills for an inquiring mind (implementing the Research-Teaching Nexus (Healey and Jenkins, 2009)) to provide a critical and evidence-based reasoned argument to enhance practice, individual woman and family collaborative care planning and decision-making as well as the application to your theoretical learning and assessments.

Sustainability and climate change factor widely in the national context (Richardson et al., 2017) and will impact upon the midwifery profession and health care generally.

This resonates with contemporary health care policy locally, nationally, and internationally (Renfrew et al., 2014; Cummings and Bennett, 2012; The NHS England, 2016b; NHS, 2019; Naylor, 2019; NHS, 2020; NHS Employers, 2020). With this in mind, this resource embraces these core education values with identified reflective and professional development activities for you to complete along the way. As a future leader and change agent (Stefancyk et al., 2013) it is essential that you remain true to your values and belief systems and consider honestly where your personal blockers and facilitators lay as well as where you consider them to sit professionally at local, national, and international levels. It is when you truly open yourself up to being 'vulnerable' (Brown, 2015) that you undertake personal and professional development that is sometimes painful and other times enlightening, in order to move forward proactively. Domain 5 within the NMC (2019) standards concern you taking ownership for your own learning and development; this resource intends to support this.

The chapters can be read and re-read as you develop your skills and knowledge base. As the depth of your knowledge expands, you will view the chapters differently on re-reading and hopefully will glean more useful assistance from within. Vignettes provide an elaboration of and insight into aspects related to others' experiences linked to their own participation in case load held practices and/or continuity of carer experiences to support your thinking, skills development and planning of care using collaborative decision-making with all involved.

## Terminologies used throughout the book

The contemporary midwifery professional world is fast evolving to meet the needs of complex and ever-changing health care requirements of the public, changing telehealth technologies (Wessex Institute, 2020; Salisbury et al., 2017), workforce (Emmanuel et al., 2020; Dall'ora, 2020), societal and professional expectations, changing policy and implementation science (BioMed Central Ltd, 2020). The NMC published their new suite of education standards in 2018 (Part 1: Standards framework for nursing and midwifery and Part 2: Standards for student supervision and assessment (SSSA) culminating in 2019 with the Part 3: Standards for pre-registration midwifery programmes (that include the standards of proficiency for midwives)). The standards of proficiency for midwives are immense, to reflect the current realities of the practising midwife and future proofing the ever-expanding role of the registered midwife. They reflect the changing global world of midwifery and the impact on women's human right to health (WHO, 2020) locally, nationally, and internationally (WHO, 2019). Childbirth should be safe, transformative, and rewarding for all women and their families across the globe hence, midwifery education and practices must be set at an international standard to embrace the transient local, national, and international community thus aiming to improve overall health across the continuum of care, reducing maternal and newborn mortality and morbidity (WHO, 2019; pp. iv and vi). Terminologies equally have changed. This book aims to use the most contemporary terminologies throughout but will occasionally refer to outgoing phrases that remain common place in the practice arena amongst clinical colleagues. As such, we have used the phrase 'case load held practice' interchangeably throughout with 'continuity of carer'. This is to reflect the changing landscape whilst also being mindful that many organisations continue to use the phrases case load held practice and/or case-loading to encompass continuity of carer. Examples of changing terminologies are listed in

*Table 1.1* Examples of changing terminologies throughout practice

| Existing and changing terminology | Contemporary terminology |
|---|---|
| Case-loading/ case load held practices | Continuity of carer |
| Low risk | Universal care |
| High risk | Additional care needs |
| Mentor/sign off mentor | Practice supervisor, Practice Assessor, Academic Assessor |

Table 1.1. It is acknowledged that change in practice is slow as these new terminologies filter through and are normalised in our everyday dialect. You may still hear professionals referring to low and high-risk settings. This may remain appropriate in some instances; however, it must be stressed that all women and their newborns receive 'universal care' as standard regardless of risk status and women and newborns who have an identified risk will have 'additional care' needs. Some organisations refer to certain cohorts of women as 'needing extra support' and have geared their continuity of carer teams to address these areas. Examples of this may be women with diabetes, the Black, Asian, Minority Ethnic (BAME) communities (now also known as Black and Brown women or Black and Asian women (Morris, 2020)), migrant women, women with previous still births or infant loss, and weight management, to name but a few.

**Box 1.2 Activity 1.2**

What do these existing and new terminologies mean for you and how do these resonate with your own perceptions of health care provision?

## What is case load held practice and continuity of carer?

Case load held practice is not a new concept. It is a model of care whereby a named midwife is assigned to a small group of women to provide antenatal, intra partum and post-partum care. It is typical for a small team of midwives to work concordantly to support and cover for each other to achieve improvements in quality care and outcomes (WHO, 2020; Ford, 2013; Tracy et al., 2013) for women of any risk. Midwifery continuity of carer describes the consistency of a named midwife and/or team providing seamless care across the pregnancy continuum (NHS England, 2017a; RCM, 2018) which is known to have positive health outcomes (Sandall et al., 2016). Midwifery continuity of carer can be arranged via different models such as a case load or a team approach; the main difference being the number of women cared for as part of the case load. Typically, a midwife in a case load practice will have up to 45 women per year. This may differ dependent upon the risk and need of the women. A team approach may have up to 360 women across a small team of approximately six midwives (Mortensen et al., 2019) all known to the women within the team case load. There are many inconsistencies across the UK in relation to the interpretation of case load held practice resulting in a hybrid of models aiming to achieve the objectives of the continuity of carer philosophy. This will be considered further within Chapters 2 and 3.

Whilst many midwives agree with the concepts of continuity of carer and cannot dispute the positive health benefits, many remain wary of the potential impact upon their own well-being and ability to achieve true continuity of carer in practice (NHS Employers, 2020; Sandall, 1997; Menke et al., 2014). It is clear from the evidence presented in Chapter 3 that women and their partners have positive experiences following this model of care (Forster et al., 2016) and this book aims to capture the voices of the women and partners and midwives that experience this approach to care provision. For students at the beginning of their careers, working to the continuity of carer principles may be the norm in their practice, education and want, however it maybe that the reality is quite different. Students may want to embark on a continuity of carer path, but they are not in charge of organising and delivering a continuity project.

The NMC (2019) Standards for Pre-Registration Midwifery Programmes have set continuity of carer high on their agenda by devoting Domain 2 to develop you as a skilled and safe, compassionate, kind, empathic and trustworthy midwife of the future who has the potential to influence and change midwifery care. Your interaction with service users will help you to develop professional communication from which you can develop critical decision-making and clinical reasoning skills in partnership. This will ensure a safe approach to care and will strengthen both your own and client capabilities (NMC, 2019a; Kirkup, 2015; Robinson and Webber 2013, Tanner et al., 2017).

The recent unprecedented global pandemic (Dashraath et al., 2020) has led to continuity of carer projects and targets for implementation to be delayed in some areas. Students have also been discouraged to attend case load appointments with women due to social distancing (Willan et al., 2020) when they have been able to attend clinical practice (Health Education England, 2020). Many maternity services have cancelled case load practices and unnecessary face to face contacts to halt the spread of disease and have no immediate intention of resuming prior activities, or at least not in the same way that have previously been administered. New technological advances have rocketed, pushing the NHS into the modern telehealth era, which many predict will be the new normal. If this is the case, continuity of carer practices will equally need to continuously evolve to meet the needs and expectations of the public and national policy implementation targets. To some extent the future is less obvious, resulting in the need to be responsive and flexible to changing health needs and the need to develop resilience in dealing with the new pace of change. These realities are further deliberated throughout the chapters.

## Following a 'values based enquiry' journey

### Box 1.3 Activity 1.3

Before you progress further into the chapter, what are your values and belief systems? How do they differ depending on what context you are in, or are they the same? What was it that has shaped these values and beliefs during your lifetime? Have you had a personal experience that has changed or challenged how you perceive and view the world you inhabit? How do you feel, and respond if another person challenges your values and beliefs or has an opposing viewpoint?

It is widely acknowledged since the Lord Laming Inquiry (2009) that all health care professionals are expected to apply learning from inter-professional education to one's own professional context. More recent reports such as Francis (2013), Kirkup (2015) and Ockenden (2020) ensure that kindness and compassion remain at the fore of one's professional values, as can be witnessed throughout the NMC (2019) standards. One strategy to achieve this is through a 'values based enquiry' journey (VBE) (Kitson-Reynolds, 2020). To foster the VBE philosophy, facilitated sessions can be planned to integrate theory and practice, to promote reflective practice and to challenge yourselves and others to achieve best practice. McLean's (2012) VBE model has formed the basis of the design of a three-year journey to promote Kitson-Reynolds' most contemporary (2020) values-based concept that you can follow throughout your education and professional development (Figure 1.1). The principles of McLean's (2012) 'yellow brick road' encompass 'the head' – to think and reflect whilst using the knowledge and practical skills learnt, 'the heart' – to show care compassion, and 'the nerve' – to show courage and ability to advocate for others. The VBE concept has been applied to one AEI 'journey' and is located within the resources chapter as an example to follow.

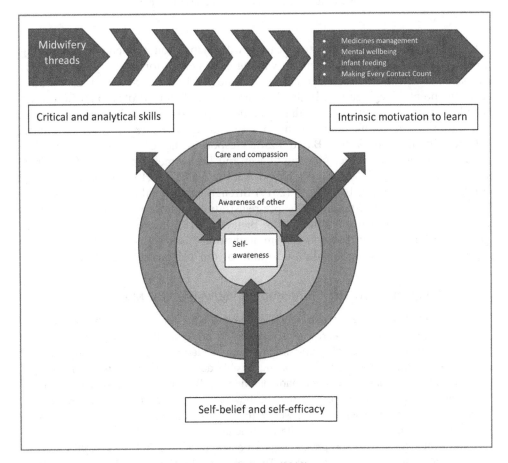

*Figure 1.1* Values based enquiry based on McLean (2012)

Table 1.2  Ten commitments (NHS England, 2016a)

| Commitment | Leading change, adding value |
|---|---|
| 1 | We will promote a culture where improving the population's health is a core component of the practice of all nursing, midwifery, and care staff |
| 2 | We will increase the visibility of nursing and midwifery leadership and input in prevention |
| 3 | We will work with individuals, families, and communities to equip them to make informed choices and manage their own health |
| 4 | We will be centred on individuals experiencing high value care |
| 5 | We will work in partnership with individuals, their families, carers, and others important to them |
| 6 | We will actively respond to what matters most to our staff and colleagues |
| 7 | We will lead and drive research to evidence the impact of what we do |
| 8 | We will have the right education, training, and development to enhance our skills, knowledge and understanding |
| 9 | We will have the right staff in the right places and at the right time |
| 10 | We will champion the use of technology and informatics to improve practice, address unwarranted variations and enhance outcomes |

A strong values-based ethos to learning will enable you to demonstrate caring through evidence of a commitment to valuing each person for whom you care. This approach will ensure confidence in confirming the good character of you, as a graduate, at the point of registration. It also has an element of Inter-Professional Education embedded within the process so that you develop a deeper understanding of the importance of inter-professional team work to enhance the care provided to women and their families. The Values Based Journey espouses the 'Compassion in Practice' (Commissioning Board Chief Nursing Officer and Department of Health (DH) Chief Nursing Adviser, 2012), 'Leading Change Adding Value' (NHS, 2016), The Lancet Series (Renfrew et al., 2014), WHO (2019) Strengthening Quality Midwifery Education' and NMC (2019) 'Standards for pre-registration midwifery programmes'. There are 6 Cs related to practice (Cummings & Bennett, 2012) – Care, Compassion, Courage, Commitment, Competence and Communication – and Ten commitments (Table 1.2) all of which act as the foundation to link to your personal care philosophy.

**Box 1.4 Vignette 1.1: The Southampton Midwifery VBE Model**

Using a strength based approach (Saleebey, 2013), there are eight sessions throughout the academic year. The VBE sessions are typically 1.5 hours maximum when conducted within small groups. It is recommended that you space these activities across your academic year. Working flexibly across the clinical maternity services, covering a 24/7 period over many differing locations is not conducive to joining together for VBEs during practice periods however, these sessions could form the basis for clinical reflective sessions with your peers, practice supervisors or practice assessors and/or Professional Midwifery Advocates.

The NMC (2019) uses the psychology principles of you having a 'strength based approach' to learning the profession. This relies on the tenets that strengths are naturally inherent within you (Saleebey, 2013) and not necessarily learnt. You bring these strengths to all that you undertake and accomplish. The strength-based approach cultivates these assets in a proactive way to develop your resilience throughout life. This has a good fit with the VBE journey whereby at the end of the journey it is expected that you realise that you have had these necessary qualities all along and that this journey has merely been you honing them. Prior to commencing care delivery, it is essential to review your own level of competency and where your limitations lay as set out within the NMC Code (2015).

### VBE – what is in it?

The VBE journey covers many agreed values that enhance the 'humanised' (Page & Creery, 2019) themes throughout your curriculum and NMC (2019) standards, and embraces both universal societal and general AEI core values e.g., learning disabilities, self-awareness, communication, cultural competence, human rights, recycling and sustainability, and the impact of midwifery on climate change. The values have been designed for the whole three-year journey linking contemporary issues within local and national practices, generic NHS England principles, political awareness and the 6 Cs (Cummings & Bennett, 2012), the Lancet Series (Renfrew et al., 2014), Morecambe bay (Kirkup, 2015), the Francis report (Francis, 2013) and the Ockenden report (Ockenden, 2020) should be covered by all groups. You are encouraged to come together for seminars to reflect, discuss, and quietly contemplate you as an individual, and to challenge yourself and others to develop your own plan for becoming the midwife you set out to be, if not more. This journey at times may become uncomfortable for your own values and belief systems, but by becoming vulnerable (Brown, 2015) you will hopefully become stronger.

## Professional Midwifery Advocates

Since changes to legislation in April 2017, your local National Health Service Maternity Services will have identified an individual or team of Professional Midwifery Advocates (PMAs) who support midwives, using the A-Equip model (NHS England, 2017a), through their professional development. This may include reviewing and facilitating the development of individual resilience, acting as the confirmer or support for revalidation (NMC, 2019b), supporting with clinically related activities such as statement writing and audit, and linking to maternity services quality improvement strategies through attendance at clinical events, and lessons learnt events.

The PMA team may comprise practising midwives across all areas of the service and University teaching team. All PMAs are available to support students in practice and you may have a designated named PMA for students. An example could be where a university employed PMA takes the lead in supporting students who have experienced an incident in clinical practice to debrief the clinical event, attend meetings, statement writing and as a support with HSIB investigations. Your university/Trust PMA may host 'Restorative Clinical Supervision (RCS)' group discussions linked to the practice experience placements and provide individual and group RCS when students individually wish to review and reflect with and without clinical colleagues (Pettit & Stephen 2015; NHS England, 2017a).

The role of the PMA will be represented within your AEI's curriculum development and through delivery of education activities. These may include focusing on what a PMA is and how they can support you through education and beyond, considering what your own professional responsibilities are, and understanding the process of Revalidation.

The new NMC (2019) Standards for pre-registration midwifery programmes, particularly Domain 5, support the development of professional safety not only for women and their newborn infants, but for each practising midwife through a 'Strength based Approach' (Saleebey, 2013) to 'Strengthen your capabilities' as a resourceful and flexible midwife needing to work in stressful and difficult situations [Standard 5.13]. The team of PMAs will support you and the wider team of midwives to build your psychological safety, foster a learning culture and understand and apply the principles of human factors when working with colleagues [Standard 5.4].

## So, what does this book have to offer?

Chapter 2 sets the political and professional context historically through to the present day typically, but not exclusively to the UK. There appears to be a healthy global respect for the truly autonomous midwifery practice that case load held practices affords midwives within the UK. This claim can be linked to increased levels of satisfaction and outcomes evidenced by research and articulated by the women and their families that have experienced this model of care. The chapter explores the success of the New Zealand Partnership Model and how the midwifery curricula has developed to support the midwife of 2030 and beyond. Case load held practice has typically been linked to groups of women requiring extra support to achieve improved health outcomes. Continuity of carer is gaining greater interest to women from ethnic backgrounds and/or those who live in poverty.

The author, Maggie O'Brien has worked in a variety of clinical settings across the UK and in Auckland, New Zealand. She has been a Director of Midwifery in both the UK and New Zealand, adapting existing maternity services in the UK and managing the interface between established midwifery continuity of care services and the acute service in New Zealand. Maggie therefore has acquired an extensive knowledge of midwifery models of care (including continuity of care models) both in the UK and New Zealand. These professional experiences are drawn upon to appropriately apply current legislation, regulation and government policy to case load practice. The implementation of Better Births: Improving outcomes of maternity services (NHS England, 2016a) including case load practice is paramount across the 4 countries of the UK. The establishment of continuity of carer will be key to implementing the urgent recommendations of the Ockenden Report (Ockenden 2020), in particular the recommendation to listen to women and their families.

The implementation of the Better Births recommendations is impacting all maternity services and midwives' working patterns. With national implementation targets set, it is high on the agenda for all clinical areas. Therefore, different models of case load held practice are considered together with the challenges they present. Whilst it is acknowledged that throughout pre-registration training, student midwives will have exposure to a plethora of experiences, the reality is that all UK students will need to be prepared following the continuity of carer philosophy whilst undergraduates, as this is most likely to be the model of care they will be employed in.

Lesley Turner considers the evidence base on case load held practice and the related health benefits that a continuity of carer and case loading model brings to women and their families in Chapter 3. The benefits to the midwife, woman and her family and maternity service delivery are considered where a continuity of carer model has already been implemented whilst taking into consideration a safe workforce perspective. Lesley has previously undertaken systematic literature reviews and is researching safe staffing in midwifery. Her previous public health teaching focusing on inequalities in health outcomes is pivotal in interpretations of data and her understanding of vulnerable groups. Lesley is a promoter of case load midwifery, due to the potential for improved physical and mental health outcomes and to improve life-chances in vulnerable groups.

Much has already been written on social inequalities and outcomes of a continuity of carer approach, such as Sandall et al. (2016), Sandall (2017) and Dawson et al. (2015), but not explicitly linked to safe staffing or linking to the student midwife and/or midwife experiences or the implementation of variants on continuity of carer models. A realistic, holistic, balanced interpretation of the evidence base is presented highlighting both strengths and limitations of student midwives and midwives working within a continuity of carer model and the potential for burnout amongst staff. The critical discussion focuses on the risks, benefits, and impact on health outcomes for women and families, linking to recent MBRRACE reports. Whilst there have been suggestions as to how a continuity of carer model might be implemented in clinical practice (RCM, 2017), there is no 'one-size fits all' approach, and this chapter aims to present an evidence informed discussion as to what continuity of carer means in your reality. The chapter concludes with recommended practicalities of how to provide case load held experience and links to Chapters 4 and 5 for realistically planning clinical placements within case load held teams for all student midwives.

We have entitled Chapter 4 practicalities: student experience of case-loading as it presents the practical tips students require to plan, implement, and evaluate for a case load held midwifery practice. Kate was Ellen's student for three years and has undertaken case load held practice as the lead carer for a minimum of five women under direct supervision of a responsible named midwife. Since qualifying, Kate has worked within a midwifery led community team, most recently providing one to one care for women needing extra support. She has used her experiences as a student to support students as a practice supervisor with their case load held experiences. Often her role highlights to student midwives the commitments required when case loading and the impact of direct and indirect promises being made around planned visits, expectations for both the student and the women, all of which are explored further in the chapter. There are typically two reactions when introducing case load experiences to students. The first is excitement to be undertaking one to one care across the pregnancy and birth continuum, and the second being one of anxiety as to how they will achieve continuity of carer when they themselves have complex issues in their own worlds such as travelling, being a single parent, being a carer, or holding a part time job to be able to complete the training programme. Through a commitment to delivering person-centred care, this chapter will equip you with the skills and knowledge to empower and strengthen the capabilities of women to take responsibility for their own health (NMC, 2019a). Continuity of carer experiences ensure that you develop effective communication skills within a multi-disciplinary team to provide safe care to meet the physical, psychological, environmental, social, emotional, and spiritual needs of women within diverse realities. Reflective activities will develop your analytical skills to debate, problem solve and make robust clinical care plans to enhance quality care within a changing health and social care environment whilst demonstrating self-management.

Chapter 5 considers practical 'tips' from the practice supervisor, practice assessor and academic assessor perspectives required to support students in planning, implementing, and evaluating case load held practices. As both academic assessor and module lead, Marie uses experiences from the setting up of case load/continuity of carer practice requirements for curriculum validation, liaising with practice partners to devise meaningful clinical experiences and reviewing themes highlighted through the moderation of case load clinical assessments and reflective course requirements to enhance the student experience of case load held practice and the experiences of the users involved. Resources commented upon in this chapter can be located as a support within the final chapter of the book and act as an aide meant to be adapted to meet the requirements of your locality.

Kate and Emer consider the emotional aspects of delivering continuity of carer in Chapter 6. They provide you with some examples about what you may expect and what the impact of case load held practice and the levels of responsibility may have on you as the individual practitioner as well as being within a wider multi-disciplinary team. Using their experiences in contemporary clinical practice both Emer and Kate consider the added 'unseen' aspects and impact of preparing and delivering continuity of carer to women on one's own work life balance and professional boundaries. These include decision-making, human factors, consideration of yours and other's professional boundaries and responsibilities, managing a work life balance when being on call and when you have other commitments inside/outside of work, how your levels of confidence waiver and how to get that important peer and professional support during the more challenging times.

Using a collective voice and range of experiences, Chapter 7 invites you to consider how to use your experiences to further your professional development. You are encouraged to use reflective practice to enhance your knowledge and understanding of continuity of carer service delivery at local and individual levels. Lifelong learning and professional requirements are components of a midwife's career to strength yours and other capabilities in an increasingly diverse and complex world of health care and maternity care. The UK profession-specific regulatory body, The Nursing and Midwifery Council, monitor and maintain a professional register of nurses and midwives who continue to demonstrate they meet the Code (NMC, 2015) through their own quality monitoring and development activities at revalidation every three years. This is achieved by incorporating the user voice into reflective practice to enhance your own care provision and the maternity services as a whole. Vignettes strengthen the understanding of reality in practice through real midwife voices and narratives.

Chapter 8 challenges you to start thinking about how you can make changes to services and how these can be evaluated to ensure they are effective in their aim and objective. Often and more historically, new concepts are introduced into clinical practice as a fait accompli, normalised within practice and never evaluated. This chapter provides you with questions to consider how you would evaluate continuity of carer practices within your practice areas using your student final year project.

Research, service evaluation, audit and quality improvement methods are introduced to you to start your critical thinking and appraisal of services for you to make change in the practice setting whilst developing your research skills. Some templates are provided in Chapter 10 that students have used to support their project planning and delivery.

Chapter 9 capitalises on the research and work that Ellen and Kate have previously undertaken surrounding supporting the transition from being a student midwife to 'becoming' a newly qualified practitioner (Kitson-Reynolds, 2010). This has been mapped against the new expectations for being ready and fit for first post. At the point of registration, if not before, you will be expected to be competent at universal care with competency at the more advanced care needs ready to fulfil the realities of being part of the clinical workforce. This chapter will set out the student midwife developing expectations versus qualified expectations from the day of your first post. Activities have been considered to help you move from dependence to independence by ensuring you have insight into the realities of the career of a midwife in a modern context through the identification of continuous professional development. Our intention is to start the process of you role modelling the practice of autonomous, professional, responsible and safe midwifery care which underpins the delivery of intelligent high quality compassionate, kind, woman-centred, evidence-based midwifery practice. This will include understanding the importance of service user involvement strategies to enhance the service (Kirkup, 2015; Offender Health Collaborative, 2015; Arnstein, 1969).

You will be introduced to the principles of revalidation (required by all midwives continuing their careers past registration) (NMC, 2019b) so that you can start to collate evidence of your professional development from the first day of your programme. You are encouraged to demonstrate an inquiring mind through reflection and lifelong learning; be self-aware; develop the knowledge and skills to ensure you are competent and confident in practice; through a strength based approach possess self-belief and have self-efficacy; will have developed the courage and character necessary to speak out and to 'make a difference' as practitioners and leaders of and within the midwifery profession. It is anticipated that by embracing technological changes, vision, and digital literacy to innovate improving health outcomes, you will have the transferable skills to enable you to become a provider of quality maternity care for women and families to manage change effectively and respond to challenging demands.

The final chapter contains practical resources such as, work sheets and 'journeys' that have been referred to within previous chapters. These resources are available to you as a template that can be adapted to be meaningful to you and your own programme of midwifery education. These are not meant to replace your AEI documentation, but complement or highlight nuances between different autonomous practicing midwives.

## References

Arnstein, S.R. (1969). A ladder of citizen participation. *JAIP*, 35(4): 216–224.

BioMed Central Ltd (2020). *Implementation Science*. Springer Nature. Available at: https://implementationscience.biomedcentral.com/ [accessed: 28th December 2020].

Brown, B. (2015). *Rising Strong*. London: Vermillion.

Ciliska, D., Thomas, H., & Buffett, C. (2010). *An Introduction to Evidence-Informed Public Health and a Compendium of Critical Appraisal Tools for Public Health Practice.* Ontario, National Collaborating Centre for Methods and Tools.

Commissioning Board Chief Nursing Officer and DH Chief Nursing Adviser (2012). *Compassion in Practice.* Leeds: Department of Health.

Cummings, J., & Bennett, V. (2012). *Compassion in Practice: Nursing, Midwifery and Care Staff our Vision and Strategy.* Leeds: Department of Health.

Dall'ora, C., Ball, J., Reinius, M., & Griffiths, P. (2020). Burnout in nursing: A theoretical review. *Human Resources for Health,* 18(1): 41.

Dashraath, P., Wong, J.L.J., Lim, M.X.K., Lim, L.M., Li, S., et al. (2020). Coronavirus disease 2019 (COVID-19) pandemic and pregnancy. *American Journal of Obstetrics and Gynecology,* 222(6): 521–531. https://doi.org/10.1016/j.ajog.2020.03.021.

Dawson, K. et al. (2015). Exploring midwifery students' views and experiences of case load midwifery: A cross-sectional survey conducted in Victoria, Australia. Available at: www.mid wiferyjournal.com/article/S0266-6138(14)00244-7/abstract [accessed: 9 September, 2020].

Department of Health (2015). *The NHS Constitution: The NHS Belongs To Us All.* Leeds: Crown Copyright.

Emmanuel, T., Dall'ora, C., Ewings, S., & Griffiths, P. (2020). Are long shifts, overtime and staffing levels associated with nurses' opportunity for educational activities, communication and continuity of care assignments: Across-sectional study. *International Journal of Nursing Studies Advances.* https://doi.org/10.1016/j.ijnsa.2020.100002.

Ford, S. (2013). Case load midwifery is safe and cost effective. *Nursing Times.* Available at: www.nursingtimes.net/roles/midwives-and-neonatal-nurses/caseload-midwifery-is-safe-and-cos t-effective-17-09-2013/ [accessed: 10 September, 2020].

Forster, D., McLachlan, H., Davey, M., Biro, M., Farrell, T., Gold, L., Flood, M., Shafiei, T., & Waldenström, U. (2016). Continuity of care by a primary midwife (case load midwifery) increases women's satisfaction with antenatal, intrapartum and postpartum care: Results from the COSMOS randomised controlled trial. *BMC Pregnancy and Childbirth,* 16(1): 28.

Francis, R. QC (2013). *Report of the Mid Staffordshire NHS Foundation Trust Public Inquiry – Executive Summary.* London: Crown Copyright.

Healey, M., & Jenkins, A. (2009). Developing students as researchers. In S.K. Haslett & H. Rowlands (eds), *Linking Research and Teaching in Higher Education.* Newport: University of Wales, pp. 7–11.

Health Education England (2020). Coronavirus (COVID-19) information for midwives. London, Health Education England. Available at: www.hee.nhs.uk/coronavirus-covid-19/ coronavirus-covid-19-information-midwives [accessed: 28 December, 2020].

Huber, U., & Sandall, J. (2006). Continuity of carer, trust and breastfeeding MIDIRS. *Midwifery Digest,* 16(4): 445–449.

International Confederation of Midwives (2017). International definition of a midwife. Geneva: International Confederation of Midwives. Available at: www.internationalmidwives.org/our-work/policy-and-practice/icm-definitions.html [accessed: 7 September, 2020].

International Confederation of Midwives Global Standards for Midwifery Education (2010 amended 2013). The education standards. Available at: www.internationalmidwives.org/wha t-we-do/education-coredocuments/global-standards-education/ [accessed: 10 December, 2019].

Kirkup, B. (2015). *The Report of the Morecambe Bay Investigation.* Preston: Morecambe Bay Investigation Copyright.

Kitson-Reynolds, E. (2010). *The Lived Experience of Newly Qualified Midwives.* Thesis, University of Southampton.

Kitson-Reynolds, E. (2020). *The University of Southampton Midwifery Values Based Enquiry Journey.* Southampton: University of Southampton.

LordLaming (2009). *The Protection of Children in England: A Progress Report*. London: The Stationary Office.

McLean, C (2012). The yellow brick road: A values based curriculum model. *Nurse Education in Practice*, 12: 159–163.

Menke, J., Fenwick, J., Gamble, J., et al. (2014). Midwives' perceptions of organisational structures and processes influencing their ability to provide case load care to socially disadvantaged and vulnerable women. *Midwifery*, 30(10): 1096–1103.

Morris, N. (2020). The BAME debate: Why terminology matters when we're talking about race. Metro.co.uk [online] Available at: https://metro.co.uk/2020/07/07/bame-debate-why-terminology-matters-when-talking-about-race-12954443/ [accessed: 28 December, 2020].

Mortensen, B., Diep L.M., Lukasse, M., et al. (2019). Women's satisfaction with midwife-led continuity of care: An observational study in Palestine. *BMJ Open*, 9: e030324. doi:10.1136/bmjopen-2019-030324.

Muzik, M., & Borovska, S. (2010). Perinatal depression: Implications for child mental health. *Mental Health in Family Medicine*, 7(4): 239–247.

Naylor, C. (2019). The NHS and climate change: A decade of distraction. Kings Fund. Available at: www.kingsfund.org.uk/blog/2019/04/nhs-climate-change [accessed: 9th September, 2020].

NHS England (2016a). Better Births: Improving outcomes of maternity services in England. National Maternity Review. Available at: www.england.nhs.uk/wp-content/uploads/2016/02/national-maternity-review-report.pdf [accessed: 14th March, 2020].

NHS England (2016b). *Leading Change Adding Value*. Leeds: NHS England.

NHS England (2017a). Implementing better births: Continuity of carer. Available at www.england.nhs.uk/publication/implementingbetter-births-continuity-of-carer [accessed: 29 November, 2020].

NHS England (2017b). A-EQUIP midwifery supervision model. Available at: https://www.england.nhs.uk/mat-transformation/implementing-better-births/a-equip/a-equip-midwifery-supervision-model/ [accessed: 28 December, 2020].

NHS England (2019). NHS Long Term Plan: Online version of the NHS Long Term Plan. London: NHS England. Available at: www.longtermplan.nhs.uk/online-version/ [accessed: 29 November, 2020].

NHS (2020). Greener NHS Campaign to tackle climate 'health emergency'. Available at: www.england.nhs.uk/2020/01/greener-nhs-campaign-to-tackle-climate-health-emergency/ [accessed: 9 September, 2020].

NHS Employers (2020). We are the NHS: People Plan 2020/21 action for us all. NHS Improvement. Available at: www.england.nhs.uk/publication/we-are-the-nhs-people-plan-for-2020-21-action-for-us-all/ [accessed: 30 December, 2020].

Nursing and Midwifery Council (2015/2018). *The Code: Standards of Conduct, Performance and Ethics for Nurses and Midwives*. London: NMC.

Nursing and Midwifery Council (2018). *Realising Professionalism: Standards for Education and Training: Part 1: Standards Framework for Nursing and Midwifery Education*. London: NMC. Available at: www.nmc.org.uk/globalassets/sitedocuments/standards-of-proficiency/standards-framework-for-nursing-and-midwifery-education/education-framework.pdf [accessed: 1 September, 2020].

Nursing and Midwifery Council (2018). *Part 2: Standards for Student Supervision and Assessment*. London: NMC.

Nursing and Midwifery Council (2019a). *Standards for Pre-Registration Midwifery programmes*. London: NMC.

Nursing and Midwifery Council (2019b). *Realising Professionalism: Standards for Education and Training*. London: NMC. Available at: https://www.nmc.org.uk/globalassets/sitedocuments/education-standards/education-framework.pdf [accessed: 1 September, 2020].

Nursing and Midwifery Council (2019c). *Revalidation*. London: NMC. Available at: http://revalidation.nmc.org.uk/ [accessed: 28 December, 2020].

Ockenden, D. (2020). *Ockenden Report. Emerging Findings and Recommendations from the Independent Review of Maternity Services at the Shrewsbury and Telford Hospital NHS Trust.* London, HMSO.

Offender Health Collaborative (2015). *Liaison and Diversion Manager and Practitioner Resource: Service User Involvement.* Leeds: NHS England.

Office for National Statistics (2019). Families and households in the UK: 2019. Available at: www.ons.gov.uk/peoplepopulationandcommunity/birthsdeathsandmarriages/families/bulletins/familiesandhouseholds/2019 [accessed: 28 December, 2020].

Page, L., & Creery, T. (2019). Humanising birth: Hope for the future even in war. *All4Maternity.* Available at: www.all4maternity.com/humanising-birth-hope-for-the-future-even-in-war/ [accessed: 28 December, 2020].

Pettit, A., & Stephen, R., (2015). *Supporting Health Visitors and Fostering Resilience Supporting Health Visitors and Fostering Resilience.* London: Institute of Health Visiting.

Royal College of Midwives (2017). The contribution of continuity of midwifery care to high quality maternity care. Available at: www.rcm.org.uk/sites/default/files/Cntinuity%20of%20Care%20A5%2012pp%202107_6.pdf [accessed: 19 February, 2019].

Royal College of Midwives (2018). *Position Statement: Midwifery Continuity of Carer* (MCOC). London: RCM.

Renfrew, M.J., McFadden, A., Bastos, M.H., Campbell, J., Channon, A.A., Cheung, N.F., et al. (2014). Midwifery and quality care: Findings from a new evidence-informed framework for maternal and newborn care. *Lancet Series on Midwifery*, 1: 1129–1145.

Ricardson, J., Grose, J., Bradbury, M., & Kelsey, J (2017). Developing awareness of sustainability in nursing and midwifery using scenario-based approach: Evidence from a pre and post educational intervention study. *Nurse Education Today*, 54: 51–55.

Robinson, K., & Webber, M. (2013). Models and effectiveness of service user and carer involvement in social work education: A literature review. *British Journal of Social Work*, 43: 925–944. doi:10.1093/bjsw/bcs025.

Saleebey, D. (ed.) (2013). *The Strengths Perspective in Social Work Practice*, 6th ed. Boston, MA: Allyn and Bacon.

Salisbury, C., O'Caitlin, A., Thomas, C., Edwards, L., Montgomery, A.A., et al. (2017). An evidence-based approach to the use of telehealth in long-term health conditions: Development of an intervention and evaluation through pragmatic randomised controlled trials in patients with depression or raised cardiovascular risk. *Programme Grants for Applied Research*, 5(1). doi:10.3310/pgfar05010.

Sandall, J. (1997). Midwives' burnout and continuity of care. *British Journal of Midwifery*, 5(2): 106–111.

Sandall, J. (2017). *The Contribution of Continuity of Midwifery Care to High Quality Maternity Care.* London: RCM.

Sandall, J., Soltani, H., Gates, S., Shennan, A., & Devane, D. (2016). Midwife-led continuity models versus other models of care for childbearing women. *Cochrane Database Syst Rev* 4: CD004667.

Stefancyk, A., Hancock, B., & Meadows, M.T. (2013). The nurse manager: Change agent, change coach? *Nursing Administration Quarterly*, 37(1): 13–17. doi:10.1097/NAQ.0b013e31827514f4.

Tanner, D., Littlechild, R., Duffy, J., & Hayes, D. (2017). 'Making it real': Evaluating the impact of service user and carer involvement in social work education. *British Journal of Social Work*, 47, 467–486. doi:10.1093/bjsw/bcv121.

Tapper, J. (2019, 10 March). All under one roof: The rise and rise of multigenerational life. *The Guardian.* Available at: www.theguardian.com/society/2019/mar/10/rise-of-multigenerational-family-living [accessed: 28 December, 2020].

Tracy, S.K., Hartz, D.L., Tracy, M.B., Allen, J., Forti, A., Hall, B et al. (2013). Case load midwifery care versus standard maternity care for women of any risk: M@NGO, a randomised controlled trial. *The Lancet*, 382(9906): 1723–1732.

Wessex Institute (2020). *Digital Health Research*. Southampton: University of Southampton.

WHO (2020). The case for midwifery. Available at: www.who.int/maternal_child_adolescent/top ics/quality-of-care/midwifery/case-for-midwifery/en/ [accessed: 10 September 2020].

WHO (2019). *Strengthening Quality Midwifery Education for Universal Health Coverage 2030: Framework for Action?* Geneva: WHO.

Willan, J., King, A.J., Jeffery, K., & Bienz, N. (2020). Challenges for NHS hospitals during Covid-19 epidemic. *The British Medical Journal*, 368: m1117. doi:10.1136/bmj.m1117.

# 2 Case load held practice and the national and international political/professional context

*Maggie O'Brien*

## Introduction

This chapter sets the historical and current political and professional context to case load held practice. It provides a global perspective through looking at models such as the 'Midwifery Partnership' model in New Zealand (NZ) (Guilliland & Pairman, 1995) and looks at how this model has been sustained for nearly thirty years. A comparison of the NZ model's success to the United Kingdom's (UK) implementation of the recommendations of the *Changing Childbirth Report* (Department of Health (DH), 1993) ensues. As National Health Service (NHS) Trusts in the UK work towards implementing continuity of carer models, a consideration of how these factors may affect your future practice as a midwife is presented. An exploration of how midwifery curricula are developed in NZ to equip future midwives to provide continuity of carer along with the challenges this may present to both UK Approved Education Institutions (AEIs) and NHS Trusts if continuity of carer is to be successfully implemented in line with the recommendations of the national maternity review *Better Births: Improving Outcomes of maternity services in England* (National Health Service England (NHSE), 2016) and the *NHS Long Term Plan* (2019).

## Political and historical context in the United Kingdom

Throughout history midwives have been 'with women' (Verluysen, 1980) with references to midwives evident as far back as biblical times (Exodus 1:16). Undoubtedly, up until the 1950s, midwives would have provided continuity of care, in some way, to the women for whom they cared.

> **Box 2.1 Activity 2.1**
>
> Before we explore how and when midwifery care became fragmented and the efforts that have been made in more recent times to restore continuity, take a moment to consider if you believe that the inherent 'with woman' role of the midwife is to provide continuity of midwifery carer?

So, you may be asking, what happened, how did the midwifery care we currently provide become so fragmented? To answer this question, it is only necessary to look as far back as the introduction of the NHS on 5 July, 1948. The implementation of the

DOI: 10.4324/9781003051527-2

National Health Service Act (1946) by Aneurin Bevin's post war Labour Government reorganised all maternity services to come under the management of regional hospital boards. As a result, midwifery care began to become fragmented between hospital midwives and community midwives. Not only did this change cause a fragmented maternity service, it also reinforced the medical status of pregnancy and birth (Henley-Einion, 2003). The gradual move of home birth to hospital birth for all women, no matter whether they had complications or not, occurred across the UK, under the belief that hospital birth was safer than home birth for all women (Tew, 1989).

Jean Donnison (1988) devoted the final chapter of her book 'Midwives and Medical Men; A history of the struggle for the Control of Childbirth', to describe the 'medical model' that existed in the 1980s, using examples of increasing interventions and a 'new obstetrics' that included active management of labour (O'Driscoll et al., 1973), an increasing use of machinery, fragmentation of care with the belief that women who requested a 'natural' birth were emotionally unstable and not to be taken seriously (Donnison, 1988).

Majorie Tew published a ground breaking book in 1989, *Safer Childbirth? A Critical History of Maternity Care*, that challenges the necessity for all women to give birth in hospital, together with the medicalisation and organization of the maternity services. At the same time, experts began to examine the evidence available and the National Childbirth Trust (NCT) and the Association for Improvements in Maternity Services (AIMS) began to campaign and lobby on behalf of women. In 1990–1991 growing pressure from the NCT, AIMS and midwives resulted in the House of Commons, under its chairman Nicholas Winterton, undertaking an enquiry into the maternity services in the UK, resulting in the production of the *Winterton Report* (DH, 1992). Recommendations from this report included the implementation of woman-centred maternity services, with the midwife as the central care provider. In response to the Winterton Report, Baroness Julia Cumberledge was appointed to chair an expert committee that resulted in the publication of the *Changing Childbirth Report* (DH, 1993) which if successfully implemented within the allotted five-year time frame would have radically improved maternity services to give women more choice, *continuity* and control.

The recommendations of the *Changing Childbirth Report* (DH, 1993) were embraced by many midwives who were keen to change the fragmented model of maternity care, put women at the centre of care and reduce medicalisation. Pilot sites were established, resulting in some successful schemes being implemented, including the 'Know your Midwife Scheme' (Flint, 1993) at St Georges Hospital, Tooting, London and One to One Midwifery at Queen Charlotte's Hospital, Hammersmith, London (Page, 2003). However, some midwives believed that the change to their lives was too great and the on call commitment caused stress and burn out (Sandall, 1997). This division in the midwifery profession continues today and possible reasons for this will be discussed later in the chapter. Despite studies to prove that continuity of carer improves maternal satisfaction and outcomes (Page et al., 2001: Page et al., 1999) most of these schemes have been disbanded, mainly due to lack of financial support, with no extra funding being given by the Department of Health to implement the recommendations of the *Changing Childbirth Report* (DH, 1993). The effect of starting continuity of carer projects, that of improved maternal satisfaction and clinical outcomes, then to have them disbanded due to austerity measures has had a detrimental effect on the morale of midwives resulting in many of them becoming reluctant to commit to developing further schemes. For this reason, the successful implementation of the recommendations of *Better Births: Improving Outcomes of maternity Services in England* (NHS England, 2016) and the *NHS Plan* (2019) is crucial if the morale of midwives is to be maintained and continuity of carer across the continuum of care, for most women, is achievable in the UK.

There was limited implementation of the recommendations of the *Changing Childbirth Report* (DH, 1993) across maternity services in NHS Trusts across the UK. It would depend upon where a woman lived in the UK, as to whether a local scheme existed and whether she had access to it. Austerity measures, introduced from 2009 onwards, involved cuts in staffing across the NHS as well as there being an increased ageing midwife population (leading to retirement) and midwifery profession attrition; culminating in a shortage of 2,500 midwives by 2019 (Royal College of Midwives (RCM), 2019), meaning that it became increasingly difficult to implement continuity of carer schemes.

Concerns regarding quality of care across the NHS were raised in 2013 following a public enquiry, by Robert Francis QC, into serious failings at Mid Staffordshire NHS Foundation Trust (Mid Staffordshire NHS Foundation Trust Public Inquiry, 2013). This inquiry was closely followed by an independent investigation into systematic failings of the maternity and neonatal services at the University Hospitals of Morecombe Bay NHS Foundation Trust. This investigation found twenty instances of significant failures that may have led to the deaths of three mothers and sixteen babies (Kirkup, 2015). Both investigations raised similar concerns, with the *Kirkup Report* (Kirkup, 2015) recommending a national review of the provision of maternity care. Therefore, Baroness Julia Cumberledge was again asked to independently lead a major review of maternity services across the country. The scope of this review was to assess the current maternity care provision and consider how services should be developed to meet the changing needs of women and babies (NHS England, 2016). The resulting report 'Better Births, Improving outcomes of maternity services in England' (NHS England, 2016; NHS England, 2017) concluded that despite the increase in the number of births and the increasing complexity of clinical cases, the quality and outcomes of maternity services had improved significantly over the last decade. It also highlighted significant differences between maternity care provision across the country with further opportunities to improve the safety of care for women and their families and reduce stillbirth rates (Cumberledge, 2016). The report made recommendations for improvement of maternity services to five areas, these are:

1    Personalised care
2    Continuity of Carer
3    Safer Care
4    Better postnatal and perinatal mental health
5    Multi-professional working

The recommendations regarding continuity of carer are:

i    To ensure safe care based on a relationship of mutual trust and respect in line with the woman's decision.
ii    Every woman should have a midwife, who is part of a small team of four to six midwives, based in the community who knows the women and family, and can provide continuity throughout the pregnancy, birth and postnatally.

iii Each team of midwives should have an identified obstetrician who can get to know and understand their service and can advise on issues as appropriate.

iv The woman's midwife should liaise closely with obstetric, neonatal and other services ensuring that she gets the care she needs and that it is joined up with the care she is receiving in the community.

---

**Box 2.2 Activity 2.2**

Above is the definition of continuity of carer defined within the *Better Births: Improving outcomes of maternity services in England* (NHS England, 2016), would you consider providing continuity as part of a small team of 4 to 6 midwives as described here? What do you think are the benefits for the midwife practising in this way and what would be the drawbacks?

---

The *NHS Long Term Plan* (2019) supports the recommendations of the *Better Births: Improving outcomes of maternity Services in England* (NHS England, 2016) including Maternity Transformation Programmes with enhanced and targeted continuity of care models to achieve improved outcomes. However, as with the implementation of the recommendations of the *Changing Childbirth Report (1993)* and the *Better Births: Improving outcomes of maternity services in England* (NHS England, 2016) no extra resources were or have been available to assist with implementation.

In 2017 Jeremy Hunt, the former Secretary of Health for Health and Social Care, instructed NHS Improvement to commission a review assessing the quality of investigations relating to newborn, infant and maternal harm at The Shrewsbury and Telford NHS. An initial review has been undertaken into 250 maternity cases and since 2017 many more families came forward, when complete the review will have encompassed 1,862 families; the largest clinical review in the history of the NHS (Ockenden, 2020). The initial review has resulted in the publication of the *Ockenden Report. Emerging Findings and Recommendations from the Independent Review of Maternity Services at the Shrewsbury and Telford Hospital NHS Trust* (Ockenden, 2020). Seven emerging themes and actions have been identified with local actions for learning and Immediate and Essential Actions for the Shrewsbury and Telford NHS Trust and the wider maternity system. Many of the identified seven areas for immediate essential action have already been recommended for improvement in previous reports, these are:

1 Enhanced safety
2 Listening to women and their families
3 Staff training and working together
4 Managing complex pregnancy
5 Risk assessment throughout pregnancy
6 Monitoring fetal wellbeing
7 Informed consent

Additionally, Ockenden (2020) identified a lack of kindness and compassion:

One of the most disappointing and deeply worrying themes that has emerged is the reported lack of kindness and compassion from some members of the maternity team at the Trust. Healthcare professionals are in a privileged position caring for women and their families at a pivotal time on their lives. Many of the cases reviewed have tragic outcomes where kindness and compassion is even more essential. The fact that this had found to be lacking on many occasions is unacceptable and deeply concerning.

(Ockenden, 2020, p. 11)

The lack of compassion identified within the Ockenden Report (2020), has been recognised as a concern and documented as a problem within maternity services, since 1996 (Astrup, 2015; Gillen et al., 2004; Ball et al., 2002; Hadikin & O'Driscoll, 2000). The first significant publication, by the RCM, *In Place of Fear: Recognising and Confronting the Problem of Bullying In Midwifery* (RCM, 1996) was published with the intention of raising awareness of the lack of compassion within the midwifery workforce. The RCM also commissioned research resulting in the many publications of Ball et al., (2002) and Curtis et al. (2003, 2006a, 2006b, 2006c, 2006d, 2006e, 2006f), all published with the intention of raising awareness of the problem, the detrimental effects this had on midwives and in some instances the women they provided midwifery care for. Despite this campaign to raise awareness of the issue, a research study by Gillen et al. (2009) provided conclusive evidence that bullying within the midwifery workforce still existed and to a lesser extent in midwifery education within universities, highlighting the permissive midwifery culture that allowed bullying to occur. Although these reports and publications highlight a problem within the midwifery workforce, this behaviour is sometimes reflected in the midwifery care provided to women and their families, this is evident from the findings of the investigations and published reports into maternity services over the last fifteen years. The different models of continuity of carer and the challenges associated with them will be discussed later in this chapter, however a positive midwifery culture is essential if these models are to be successfully implemented.

Following the publication of the *Mid Staffordshire NHS Foundation Trust Public Inquiry* (2013) and the *Kirkup Report* (2015), both identifying a lack of compassion, Byrom & Downe (2015) compiled and edited the book *Roar Behind the Silence. Why Kindness, Compassion and Respect Matter in Maternity Care*, reflecting their philosophical belief that kindness and compassion are fundamental to good quality maternity care. This significant book became popular on an international basis and triggered *Roar* events that explored examples of compassionate midwifery care. However, despite many midwives embracing the need to change, evidence of the continuing lack of compassion, was provided in 2016 by the RCM, through an online survey entitled 'Why midwives leave revisited' (RCM, 2016). They received 2,719 responses with the two main reasons for midwives leaving, or thinking of leaving, being poor staffing levels and the inability to provide the quality of care the midwives wanted to give. However, 19% of the midwives who had already left gave bullying from colleagues as the main reason for leaving and 11% gave bullying from a manager as the reason. Sadly, the findings of the recently published *Ockenden Report* (2020) reflect the lack of compassion researched, highlighted and discussed over, at least the last 25 years.

You may be asking yourself why so many maternity service reports, some of which are detailed above, have been written and yet the recommendations failed to be implemented, resulting in harm to women and babies (Ockenden, 2020; Kirkup, 2015). This is however only partly true, it is important to note that Baroness Cumberlege found a significant difference in the provision of maternity services across the country (NHS England, 2016). Many maternity units have successfully improved the culture within their units and implemented excellent continuity of carer models, these NHS Trusts must be recognised and commended. Where NHS Trusts have a supportive, inclusive culture with compassionate leadership the implementation of continuity of carer models will be possible, where the culture is intimidating, hierarchical with autocratic leadership it will be much more difficult. If the recommendations of *Better Births: Improving Outcomes of maternity Services in England* (NHS England, 2016), including meeting the targets for the implementation of continuity of carer, and the *Ockenden Report* (2020) are to be successfully implemented it will be crucial to draw a metaphorical line in the sand and make unkindness of all forms completely unacceptable across all maternity services.

Ironically, if the recommendations of the *Better Births: Improving Outcomes of maternity Services in England* (NHS England, 2016) are implemented across the country and continuity of carer becomes a possibility for all women, the implementation of the *Ockenden Report* (2020) recommendations are more achievable. Research demonstrates that quality of care, clinical outcomes and maternal satisfaction improve when women receive continuity of carer (Sandall, 2017; Sandall et al., 2016; Page, 2003; Page et al., 2001; Page et al., 1999), issues all identified as a concern in the *Ockenden Report* (2020)

The recently launched new Nursing and Midwifery Council (NMC) *Standards of Proficiency for Midwives* (NMC, 2019) support the recommendations of the *Better Births: Improving outcomes of maternity services in England* (NHS England, 2016) by creating Domain 2: Safe and effective midwifery care: promoting and providing continuity of care and carer:

> Midwives promote continuity of care, and work across the continuum from pre-pregnancy, pregnancy, labour and birth, postpartum, and the early weeks of newborn infants' life.
>
> (NMC, 2019, p. 16)

By making this requirement explicit in the midwifery standards the implementation of continuity of care/carer models will be easier to achieve, with each midwife now being required to demonstrate how they meet this standard.

The RCM support the principle of continuity of carer (RCM, 2018; RCM, 2017) and their involvement is essential in the implementation of new continuity of care models. The RCM has both a professional and Trade Union function, being the first professional organization to affiliate with the Trade Union Congress (TUC), an organization who lobby actively for equality and employment rights (RCM, 2020). This dual professional/trade union function of the RCM has been the subject of many debates at RCM conferences and meetings, one argument being that it is a conflict of interest for the RCM, with the other side of the argument being that having representatives who are midwives and able to understand the professional arguments provide much better outcomes when negotiating for its members.

An example of how this dual function works would be when an NHS Trust intends to implement a continuity of carer scheme and the RCM represents a midwife member who is unable to undertake the on-call hours required to fulfil the continuity of carer commitment required of them. Professionally, the RCM, would support the NHS Trust implementing the scheme, and as a Trade Union would negotiate for the members who are not able to undertake on-call commitments. Usually a resolution is achieved on behalf of the member that does not compromise the implementation of the new model of care. Other Trade Unions do not have a professional function, representing members by negotiating and bargaining with employers when workers are unhappy with pay or working conditions. Therefore they are able to oppose the implementation of continuity of carer schemes, on behalf of their midwife members without taking the professional aspects into consideration. This can sometimes have the effect of stopping the implementation of continuity of care models.

With the recommendations of the *Better Births: Improving outcomes of maternity services in England* (NHS England, 2016) combined with launch of the *Standards of Proficiency for Midwives* (NMC, 2019) the support of the RCM (RCM, 2018) and an increasing amount of research (Sandall, 2017, Sandall et al., 2016), there is now a great opportunity to improve the outcomes and experience for all women, in particular those from ethnic backgrounds and/or those living in deprived areas (Rayment-Jones et al., 2015). With the Covid 19 global pandemic some maternity services have stopped their continuity of care provision, including pilots/projects during this difficult time and some have continued with the implementation of their plans and even increased the momentum. We have seen, with the pandemic, that it is possible to achieve great change in a very short space of time; therefore it is essential now, as we emerge from the pandemic that continuity of care/carer plans are not put on hold but continue to be implemented across the country.

## Global, historical and political perspective

The hospitalization and subsequent medicalization of maternity care together with decreasing midwifery autonomy followed a similar path in NZ (Donley, 1986) as it did in the UK. During the late 1980s midwives, feminist and childbirth activists became increasingly vocal about the increasing medicalization of childbirth (Papps & Olssen, 1988). In 1990, a powerful, combined political campaign was successful in changing the law to enable midwives to practice autonomously; this political alliance of women with midwives was the foundation of NZ's model of Midwifery Partnership (Guilliland & Pairman, 2010). The 'Midwifery Partnership' model soon became internationally acclaimed as one of the most successful and autonomous models of midwifery practice (Pairman, 2006; Hendry, 2009), enabling a large majority of women in NZ to receive midwifery-led continuity of care throughout the antenatal, labour and postnatal periods for nearly thirty years, and most importantly is not only sustained but moving from strength to strength. NZ is the only country where every pregnant woman, through legislation, is entitled to continuity of maternity carer and to choose the midwife, or doctor who provides it.

When considering the lack of progress made with the implementation of the recommendations of the *Changing Childbirth Report* (DH, 1993) and subsequent reports, in the UK, a question that needs to be asked is 'How has the NZ Partnership Model of midwifery care, enabling a majority of women to receive continuity of carer, been successfully implemented and sustained for nearly 30 years?' This question will be considered by looking at legislative and regulatory differences between the two NZ and UK models of midwifery care.

Midwifery care in NZ, is nationally funded, based on Primary Care and the principles of the Partnership Model. This model is defined by Gulliland & Pairman (1995) as a relationship of 'sharing' between the women and midwife, which involves trust, shared control and responsibility with shared meaning through mutual understanding. Gilkison et. al (2013) describe the successful midwifery model as underpinned by the three pillars of education, practice and autonomy.

The principles of the NZ Midwifery Partnership Model (Gulliland & Pairman, 1995):

i   Link the needs of women and midwives together.
ii  Encourages a relationship of sharing between woman and midwife that involves trust.
iii Has shared control and decision making between the woman and the midwife.
iv  Is based on negotiation.
v   Has shared responsibility and understanding.

NZ maternity services integrate primary, secondary and tertiary services with its midwives choosing to practice as Lead Maternity Carers (LMC) or to be employed by the District Health Boards as 'core midwives'. As core midwives they usually work shifts and care for women who are admitted with complex needs and support the LMCs. In 2017, 94.2% of women chose to give birth with an LMC and 92.3% of LMCs are midwives (Ministry of Health, 2017). This means that 94.2% of women received continuity of carer over the childbirth continuum. LMCs are contracted to the Ministry of Health and are paid directly by them, meaning they are not obligated to provide maternity care to a particular maternity service. The LMCs have universal right of access to hospitals for midwives, women and babies when specialist obstetric care is required. Auckland has three main secondary/tertiary maternity units plus birth centres, meaning that a midwife has access to all three hospitals if she wishes, enabling the woman to have the choice of home birth, birth in a birth centre or secondary maternity hospital. This is only possible because NZ has a no fault medical insurance scheme which covers medical negligence claims, the LMC midwives are accountable to the NZ Midwifery Council and the Health and Disability Commissioner at the Health and Disability Commission (Health and Disability Commissioner, 2020). If the UK decided to implement a similar continuity of carer scheme as NZ, with informed choice available for all women as regards place of birth and health care practitioner it would have to be possible for independent midwives to access indemnity insurance.

The introduction of the Nurses Amendment Act in 1990 changed the law in NZ to provide a legislative framework, as described above which laid the foundation for the midwifery Partnership Model. Currently all LMCs are contracted to the Ministry of Health (2007) under Section 88 of the Public Health and Disability Act 2000 where the requirement to provide continuity of care is enshrined in legislation. It states under Part D 'The aim of lead maternity care is to provide a woman with **continuity of care** throughout pregnancy, labour and birth and the postnatal period' and that 'services are provided in a manner which supports and promotes **continuity of care**'. The fact that legislation supports midwives to provide continuity of care means that it can never be discontinued due to financial pressures, as has happened with many continuity of care schemes in the UK.

In 1990, following the legislative changes, the midwives were regulated by the Nursing Council of NZ, this changed in 2003 when the Midwifery Council of NZ was established as the regulatory authority for midwives. The principles of the Partnership Model are strictly adhered to by the Midwifery Council of NZ; since 1991 they have made it very clear that midwives are expected to work in partnership with women and that continuity of carer is central to this partnership. The first competency for entry to the Register of Midwives is described in Figure 2.1.

The NZ College of Midwives (NZCOM) is a professional organisation for midwives whose mission is to 'provide and promote quality standards for NZ Midwives. Our role is a midwifery voice for midwives and women' (NZCOM, 2020). There is a separate Trade Union called Midwifery Employee Representative and Advisory Service (MERAS). NZCOM are closely aligned to the NZ Midwifery Council and organise each midwife to have a two-yearly midwifery standards review. This is a recertification process where every midwife attends a maternity standards review consisting of another midwife and a consumer representative both trained in the review process. At the midwifery standards review each midwife:

(I)   Presents her birth outcome statistics.
(II)  Discusses her practice and ongoing education plans.
(III) Reflects on her practice against the standards of the profession.
(IV)  Provides feedback from mothers/families on the care given.

If a midwife does not attend or does not demonstrate that she has met the standards she is not able to practice. There is considerable involvement of consumer representatives in the midwifery standards review with all women involved with maternity services encouraged to complete a feedback form, which are returned directly to NZCOM. These forms are collated and discussed with the midwives at their midwifery standards review. All midwives are required to demonstrate how they 'promote and

---

The Midwifery Council of NZ Competency One for Entry to the Register of Midwives is:

"The midwife works in partnership with the woman/wahine throughout the maternity experience."

The word midwife has an inherent meaning of being "with woman". The midwife acts as a professional companion to promote each woman's right to empowerment to make informed choices about her pregnancy, birth experience and early parenthood.

The midwifery relationship enhances the health and well-being of the woman/wahine, the baby/tamaiti and their family/whanau.

The onus is on the midwife to create a functional partnership. The balance of "power" within the partnership fluctuates but it is always understood that the woman/wahine has control over her own experience.

Performance Criteria The midwife:

1.1 centres the woman/wahine as the focus of care;

1.2 **promotes and provides or supports continuity of midwifery care**

---

*Figure 2.1* Competency one for entry to the NZ register of midwives

provides or supports continuity of midwifery care' (NZCOM, 2020). Students are aware of this standard that they are required to meet from the point of qualification. All midwives are expected to hold a case load, including educators, researchers and managers, albeit a small one. The culture of providing continuity of carer is embedded as part of midwifery practice from the moment a student enters University.

---

**Box 2.3 Vignette 2.1: Jude Cottrell, New Zealand Lead Maternity Carer**

I was a young, newly trained midwife when the new system came in nearly 30 years ago, I never worked under the old system. There was a massive rejigging of the old system with a lot of up skilling. Prior to this everyone was also a nurse and I was in the first group to have taken a midwifery degree so there was a double change. There was a lot of debate and discussion about what autonomy meant, there was tension about money and also tension between the hospital and LMC midwives.

The LMC is either the GP or the midwife, the woman chooses who this will be. Under Section 88 the payment from the Ministry of Health is the same, to either the GP or midwife. At first there was a lot of resentment from the GPs as they believed care should be to the whole family, plus they lost their maternity care payment as this went to whoever provided the maternity care.

As student midwives it all depended on who your mentor was, good mentorship was the most important thing. As newly qualified midwives we were encouraged to go out as LMCs straight away as 'good to go'. Now there is an excellent first year of practice programme with mentors paid appropriately to recognise the responsibility. The LMC midwives are not paid extra to have student midwives working with them and most of them enjoy having students. In the final year there is a long block of continuity of care and students are on call for 3 months at a time and births are the priority. This way they learn what it is actually like to be on call for months at a time. The midwife stands back in the student's third year and the student learns to navigate midwifery care with the woman.

For the midwife, autonomy is decision making with the ability to balance all the family, spiritual, mental health and risk factors with the legislation behind us that stands to support and honor the women's choice without being fear or risk based.

---

As has been identified above, the success factors ensure the success of the NZ model of maternity care are:

(I) Midwifery autonomy, established since the change to legislation in 1991.
(II) Totally separate Ministry of Health funding for LMCs and acute maternity hospital services, which means that the acute service has no managerial jurisdiction over the work of the LMCs. This is significant because LMCs can plan their day and not be called to staff acute services.
(III) The requirement to provide continuity of care is enshrined in legislation.
(IV) A requirement for the midwife to provide continuity of care is part of the NZ Midwifery Council's competencies required to enter the register and practice as a registered midwife.
(V) There is a no fault medical insurance scheme.
(VI) There is strong partnership working with women, even to the extent of a user representative being part of every midwives' two-yearly Maternity Service Review.

## Case load held practice and the Midwifery Curriculum

Additional to the success factors described above is the development of midwifery education and curriculum to support midwifery autonomy, midwifery led care and the provision of continuity of carer (Pairman, 2010). Following the legislative changes in 1990, a three-year direct entry midwifery bachelor's programme was introduced in 1992, designed to prepare midwives for autonomous practice, with the first graduates registering in 1994. A growing belief that more clinical practice within the midwifery curriculum was necessary led to the NZ Midwifery Council undertaking a review of midwifery education in 2006 (Midwifery Council of New Zealand, 2007a). This resulted in a revision of the standards for approval of pre-registration midwifery education programmes resulting in a longer programme, the equivalent of four years, with increased clinical practice hours (Midwifery Council of New Zealand, 2007b). The current requirements of the NZ Midwifery Council (Midwifery Council of New Zealand, 2015) include a minimum of a total of 4800 hours, a flexible delivery approach with specific theory and practice components, including at least 2400 practice hours and 1920 theory hours. The total hours equate to four academic years but the degree is delivered over three calendar years to enable the students to maximise experimental learning opportunities across the whole year (Gilkison et al., 2015). The UK NMC sets out the standards for midwifery education in the *Standards framework for nursing and midwifery education* (NMC, 2019) and has similar requirements to the standards set by the NZ Midwifery Council; the minimum hours required are 4600 with 50% theory hours and 50% clinical hours. Both midwifery councils require students to demonstrate competency to practice and students are assessed against competencies in practice. For newly qualified midwives NZCOM run a Midwifery First Year of Practice programme, which is a funded, structured and individualised programme of one-to-one formal mentoring, education and professional development (Dixon et al., 2014). All newly qualified midwives are part of the programme whether they are an LMC or core midwife and midwives are paid to be a mentor as part of this programme. The Midwifery First Year of Practice programme means that a midwife can become an LMC at the point of qualification and know that she will be supported in practice. If the recommendations of *Better Births: Improving Outcomes of Maternity Services in England* (NHS England, 2016) are to be fully implemented newly qualified midwives will be entering continuity of care schemes and consideration will need to be given as to how these midwives will be supported in these settings, in a way that is consistent across the UK.

The difference in the NZ and UK midwifery curricula is the opportunity for every student to work in a continuity of care midwifery model for a long period of time, no matter which part of the country they are in or which University they attend. In the first two years the students work alongside a number of LMCs in the community and hospital settings so they can experience midwife-led continuity of care across the scope of practice in all settings. The most significant difference is in the final year when practice experience increases to 80% and the student midwife practices continuity of care with an LMC midwife for at least a period of nine months. This experience is invaluable and inevitably has contributed to the continuing success of the model and a contributing factor with 48% of students entering continuity of care practice at the point of qualification (Pairman et al., 2016). It provides the student with an understanding of being on call for a long period of time and how this would affect their lives as an LMC midwife. Currently many UK NHS Trusts provide limited and very different continuity of care opportunities for student midwives and these experiences are explored later in the book, however as and when the recommendations of *Better Births: Improving outcomes of maternity services in England* (NHS England, 2016) are implemented the curricula and the continuity of care experience of UK student midwives will be required to become innovative and flexible to give them opportunities to practice in this way.

## Models of continuity of carer in the UK

The fact that NZ has a clearly defined model of midwifery care that is evident to all women, midwives and student midwives and available to all women no matter their postal address is discussed above as one reason for the success and sustainability of the NZ model. Importantly all students are aware they will be required to provide continuity of care for a sustained period as a student midwife and then practice as either an LMC and provide one model of continuity of care across the continuum of midwifery practice, or as a 'core midwife', once they register as a midwife. The same consistency does not exist across the UK with very different models of continuity of carer provided by NHS Trusts. Different models of continuity of carer have existed since the recommendations of the *Changing Childbirth Report* (DH, 1993). This was an opportunity to implement a legislated model of continuity of care across the UK to meet the recommendations of the report. As discussed previously, many different models were started and subsequently stopped mainly due to lack of resources and in some cases midwives not wanting to practise in this way, in particular having on-call responsibilities. The difference in the timing between the publication of both the *Changing Childbirth Report* (DH, 1993) and *Better Births: Improving Outcomes of maternity Services in England* (NHS England, 2016) means we now have conclusive research-based evidence to support the recommendations of both reports in that continuity of carer improves both the clinical outcomes and experience for women and their families (Sandall 2017; Sandall et al., 2016; Page 2003; Page et. al., 2001; Page et al., 1999). It is important as a student midwife to be aware of the different continuity of carer models that exist and when applying for a midwifery job you ensure you apply to a maternity service that will enable you to provide continuity of carer if you want to.

When implementing a model of continuity of carer the maternity service will need to make some important decisions, these decisions will impact on how many midwives a woman will come into contact with and how you will practise as a midwife, there are no right or wrong decisions but they will impact upon clinical outcomes and the experience that a woman receives, these are:

i   Should the model include intrapartum continuity of care as well as antenatal and postnatal care? This is a significant decision because evidence suggests that models of care that provide continuity across the entire maternity episode provide improved user experience and outcomes (Sandall 2017). Including intrapartum care has been a point of contention between midwives since *Changing Childbirth Report* (DH, 1993) many of whom believe that a woman does not mind who cares for her as long as the midwife is kind and competent.

ii   Should the whole service move to a continuity of care model and operate in a similar way to the NZ model with the maternity unit staffed with a 'core staff' with the continuity of carer midwives moving in and out of the hospital with the women they care for? If this model is decided upon the most important decision is how many midwives within the service would provide continuity of care and how many would practise as part of the core team. Staffing is discussed later in the book (Chapter 3) but there must be a safe service and high risk areas need to be staffed to a high level of safety. Equally the size of a midwives caseload cannot be too high or the midwives will burn out. With the NZ model the midwife can determine the size of her caseload resulting in some midwives choosing as many as 60 women per year, which does cause them to become tired and more liable to burn out.

iii  If a percentage of the maternity service move to a continuity of care model, which group/groups of women will receive continuity of care? Should this be women who have medical conditions, for example diabetes, or women who have social complexity? There is evidence that continuity of carer significantly improves outcomes for women from ethnic backgrounds and those living in deprived areas. Therefore, if continuity of care were introduced across the UK for all women who are from ethnic backgrounds and/or those living in deprived areas (Rayment-Jones et al., 2015) there is potential to have future significant impact on women's public health including improving perinatal mental health and breast feeding rates.

iv   The recommendations of the *Better Births: Improving Outcomes of maternity Services in England* (NHS England, 2016) are that continuity of carer should be provided by a team of 4–6 midwives, therefore the following decisions will be necessary;

a    Will there be continuity of care in that one midwife will provide all care, where possible, with the support of the team or of one particular 'partner' within the team? This is the NZ model of care.

b    Will there be a continuity of carer accountability where each woman gets to know each member of the Team and there is a possibility that she will be cared for by any member of the Team available on that day.

c    How many midwives will be in the team?

d    Will there be a designated team 'leader'?

## In summary

As you can see there are many possible models of continuity of care/carer that you should be aware of, that would all impact differently on your midwifery practice. An important factor that may impact upon your practice (as discussed previously) and can affect the implementation of continuity of care/carer models is the culture within the maternity unit that provides it. Where there is a lack of compassion and where continuity of care/carer models and a fragmented model are provided alongside each other there is potential for conflict. It is therefore important there are respectful relationships between all midwives and that midwives who provide continuity of care/carer are well supported within their maternity units.

There are many midwives who are successfully improving clinical outcomes and experience, for many women across the UK, by providing midwifery continuity of care/carer, despite the current challenges that exist. However, currently whether a women receives continuity of care/carer will largely depend upon her postcode, therefore this chapter has looked at how political, historical and professional perspectives have affected the implementation of continuity of midwifery care/carer both in the UK and NZ and explored how these perspectives could influence the implementation of the recommendations of *Better Births: Improving Outcomes of maternity Services in England* (NHS England, 2016) for all women across the UK.

# References

Astrup, J. (2015). Bullying: The writing's on the wall. *Midwives*. London: Royal College of Midwives. Available at: www.rcm.org.uk/tags/midwives-magazine [accessed: 13 September, 2020].

Ball, L., Curtis, P., & Kirkham, M. (2002). *Why do Midwives Leave?* London: Royal College of Midwives.

Byrom, S., & Downe, S. (2015). *The Roar behind the Silence. Why Kindness, Compassion and Respect Matter in Maternity Care.* London: Pinter & Martin Ltd.

Cumberledge, J. (2016). *Better Births Improving Outcomes of Maternity Services in England. A Five Year Forward View for Maternity Care.* NHS England.

Curtis, P., Ball, L., & Kirkham, M. (2003). *Why do Midwives Leave? Talking to Managers.* London: Royal College of Midwives.

Curtis, P., Ball, L., & Kirkham, M. (2006a). Bullying and horizontal violence: Cultural or individual phenomena? *British Journal of Midwifery*, 14(4A): 218–221.

Curtis, P., Ball, L., & Kirkham, M. (2006b). Ceasing to practise midwifery: Working life and employment choices. *British Journal of Midwifery*, 14(6 June): 336–338.

Curtis, P., Ball, L., & Kirkham, M. (2006c). Flexible working patterns: Balancing service needs or fuelling discontent? *British Journal of Midwifery*, 14(5 May): 260–264.

Curtis, P., Ball, L., & Kirkham, M. (2006d). Working together? Indices of division within the midwifery workforce. *British Journal of Midwifery*, 14(3 March): 138–141.

Curtis, P., Ball, L., & Kirkham, M. (2006f). Why do midwives leave? (Not) being the kind of midwife you want to be. *British Journal of Midwifery*, 14(1 January): 27–31.

Curtis, P., Ball, L., & Kirkham, M. (2006e). Management and morale: Challenges in contemporary maternity care. *British Journal of Midwifery*, 14(2 February): 100–103.

Department of Health (1992). *Health Committee Second Report: Maternity Services.* London: HMSO.

Department of Health (1993). *Changing Childbirth: Report of the Expert Maternity Group Pt.1.* London: HMSO.

Dixon, L., Tumility, E., Kensington, M., Campbell, N., Lennox, S., Calvert, S., Grey, E., & Pairman, S. (2014). *Stepping Forward into Life as a Midwife on New Zealand/Aotearoa: An Analysis of the Midwifery First Year of Practice Programme 2007–2010.* Christchurch, New Zealand: New Zealand College of Midwives.

Donley, J. (1986). *Save the Midwife.* Auckland: New Woman's Press.

Donnison, J. (1988). *Midwives and Medical Men. A History of the Struggle for the Control of Childbirth*, 2nd ed. London: Historical Publications.

Flint, C., (1993). *Midwifery Teams and Case Loads.* Oxford: Butterworth Heinemann.

Gilkison, A., Giddings, L., Smythe, L. (2013). The shaping of midwifery education in Aotearoa, New Zealand. *New Zealand College of Midwives Journal*, 47: 18–23. doi:10.12784/nzcomjnl47.2013.4.18-23.

Gilkison, A., Pairman, S., McAra-Couper, J., Kensington, M., & James, L. (2015). Midwifery education in New Zealand: Education, practice and autonomy. *Midwifery*, 33. doi:10.1016/j.midw.2015.12.001.

Gillen, P., Sinclair, M., & Kernoham, G. (2004). A concept analysis of bullying in midwifery. *Evidence Based Midwifery*, 2(2): 46–51. Available at: www.rcm.org.uk/access-evidence-based-midwifery-journal [accessed: 30 December, 2020].

Gillen, P., Sinclair, M., & Kernoham, G. (2009). Student midwives' experience of bullying. *Evidence Based Midwifery*, 7(6): 46–53. Available at: www.rcm.org.uk/access-evidence-based-midwifery-journal [accessed: 30 December, 2020].

Guililand, K., & Pairman, S. (1995). *The Midwifery Partnership Model for Practice*. Wellington: Department of Nursing and Midwifery, Victoria University.

Guilliland, K., & Pairman, S. (2010). *Women's Business: The Story of the New Zealand College of Midwives 1986–2010*. Christchurch: New Zealand College of Midwives.

Hadikin, R., & O'Driscoll, M. (2000). *The Bullying Culture: Cause, Effect, Harm Reduction*. Oxford: Books for Midwives Press.

Health and Disability Commission (HDC) (2020). The Health and Disability Commissioner. Available at: www.hdc.org.nz [accessed: 6 December, 2020].

Hendry, C. (2009). The New Zealand model: A midwifery renaissance. In R.E. Davis-Floyd, B. Daviss, & J. Tritten (Eds.), *Birth Models That Work* (pp. 55–87). London: University of California.

Henley-Einion, A. (2003). The medicalisation of childbirth. In C. Squire (Ed.), *The Social Context of Birth* (pp. 55–87). Oxford: Radcliffe Publishing.

Kirkup, B. (2015). *The Report of the Morecambe Bay Investigation*. Preston: Morecambe Bay Investigation Copyright.

Mid Staffordshire NHS Foundation Trust Public Inquiry (2013). *Report of the Mid Staffordshire NHS Foundation Trust Public Inquiry: Executive Summary* [The Francis Inquiry]. London: The Stationery Office.

Midwifery Council of New Zealand (2007a). *Pre-registration Education-Summary Report*. Wellington: Midwifery Council of New Zealand.

Midwifery Council of New Zealand (2007b). *Standards for Approval of Pre-registration Midwifery Education Programmes and Accreditation of Tertiary Education Organisations*. Wellington: Midwifery Council of New Zealand.

Midwifery Council of New Zealand (2015). *Standards for Approval of Pre-registration Midwifery Education Programmes and Accreditation of Tertiary Education Organisations*, 2nd ed. Wellington: Midwifery Council of New Zealand.

*National Health Service Act* (1946). London: Stationary Office.

National Health Service England (2016). *Better Births: Improving Outcomes of Maternity Services in England. National Maternity Review*. Available at: https://www.england.nhs.uk/wp-content/uploads/2016/02/national-maternity-review-report.pdf [accessed: 14 March, 2020].

National Health Service England (2017). *Implementing Better Births: Continuity of Carer*. Available at: https://www.england.nhs.uk/publication/implementingbetter-births-continuity-of-carer [accessed: 29 November, 2020].

National Health Service England (2019). *NHS Long Term Plan: Online version of the NHS Long Term Plan*. London: NHS England. Available at: www.longtermplan.nhs.uk/online-version/ [accessed: 29 November 2020].

New Zealand College of Midwives (2020). *Midwifery Standards Review*. Available at www.midwife.org.nz/midwives/midwifery-standards-review/ [accessed: 29 November, 2020].

New Zealand Ministry of Health (2007). *Section 88 of The New Zealand Public Health and Disability Act 2000*. Available at www.health.govt.nz/system/files/documents/publications/s88-primary-maternity-services-notice-gazetted-2007.pdf [accessed: 29 November, 2020].

New Zealand Ministry of Health (2017). *Report of Maternity 2017*. Wellington, NZ: MoH.

Nursing and Midwifery Council (2019). *Standards for Pre-Registration Midwifery Programmes*. London: NMC

O'Driscoll, K., Stronge, J.M., & Minogue, M. (1973). Active management of labour. *British Medical Journal*, 3(5872): 135–137.

Ockenden, D. (2020). *Ockenden Report. Emerging Findings and Recommendations from the Independent Review of Maternity Services at the Shrewsbury and Telford hospital NHS Trust.* London: HMSO.

Page, L. (2003). One-to-one midwifery: Restoring the 'with woman' relationship in midwifery. *Journal of Midwifery & Women's Health*, 48(2): 119–125.

Page, L.A., Beake S., Vail A., McCourt C., & Hewison J. (2001). A comparative cohort study of clinical outcomes and maternal satisfaction with One-to-One Midwifery Practice. *British Journal of Midwifery*, 9(11): 700–706.

Page, L., McCourt, C., Beake, S., Hewison, J., & Vail, A. (1999). Clinical interventions and outcomes of one-to-one midwifery practice. *J Public Health Med*, 21(4): 243–248.

Pairman, S. (2006). Midwifery partnership: Working 'with' women. In L.A. Page & R. McCandlish (Eds.), *The New Midwifery: Science and Sensitivity in Practice.* Edinburgh: Elsevier.

Pairman, S. (2010). Educating midwives for autonomous practice. In K. Gulliland & S. Pairman (Eds). *Woman's Business* (pp. 480–563). Christchurch, NZ: New Zealand College of Midwives.

Pairman, S., Tumilty, L., Dixon, E., Gray, E., Campbell, N., & Calvert, S. (2016). The Midwifery First Year of Practice programme: Supporting New Zealand midwifery graduates in their transition to practice. *Journal New Zealand College Midwives*, 52: 12–19.

Papps, E., & Olssen, M. (1997). *Doctoring Childbirth and Regulating Midwifery in New Zealand: A Foucualdian Perspective.* Palmerston North: Dunmore Press.

Rayment-Jones, H., Murrells, T., & Sandall, J. (2015). An investigation of the relationship between the caseload model of midwifery for socially disadvantaged women and childbirth outcomes using routine data: A retrospective, observational study. *Midwifery*, 31(4): 409–417.

Royal College of Midwives (1996). *In Place of Fear: Recognising and Confronting the Problem of Bullying in Midwifery.* London: RCM.

Royal College of Midwives (2016). *Why Midwives Leave – Revisited.* London: RCM.

Royal College of Midwives (2017). The contribution of continuity of midwifery care to high quality maternity care. Available at: www.rcm.org.uk/sites/default/files/Cntinuity%20of%20Ca re%20A5%2012pp%202107_6.pdf [accessed: 19 February, 2019].

Royal College of Midwives (2018). *Position Statement Midwifery Continuity of Carer (MCOC).* London: RCM.

Royal College of Midwives (2019). England short of almost 2500 midwives, new birth figures confirm. Available at: www.rcm.org.uk/news-views/rcm-opinion/2019/england-short-of-alm ost-2-500-midwives-new-birth-figures-confirm/ [accessed: 19 September, 2020].

Royal College of Midwives (2020). The RCM is affiliated with the TUC. Available at: https:// www.rcm.org.uk/about-us/tuc/ [accessed: 6 December, 2020].

Sandall, J. et al. (2016). Midwife-led continuity models versus other models of care for childbearing women. *Cochrane Database Syst Rev 4*: CD004667.

Sandall, J. (1997). Midwives' burnout and continuity of care. *British Journal of Midwifery*, 5(2): 106–111.

Sandall, J. (2017). *The Contribution of Continuity of Midwifery Care to High Quality Maternity Care.* London: RCM.

Tew, M. (1989). *Safer Childbirth? A Critical History of Maternity Care.* London: Springer.

Verluysen, M. (1980). Old wives tales? Women healers in English history. In C. Davies (Ed.), *Rewriting Nursing History.* London: CroomHelm.

# 3 Evidence base on case load held practice and outcomes

*Lesley Turner*

## Introduction

This chapter considers the research evidence underpinning the introduction of case load held models. Students should be aware of both the strengths and limitations of research studies and their applicability to local practice, and should consider the possible explanations for positive outcomes associated with case load held practices. Although these are not always defined by the evidence, influencing factors such as close inter-personal relationships, disclosure, service access and communication could explain why case load held practice has been associated with improved outcomes. Readers are encouraged to reflect on the evidence as they interpret the implications for practice. Evidence of negative effects are presented, and readers are encouraged to reflect on how these effects could be mitigated when implementing case loading in practice.

This chapter is organised into five sub-sections:

1 Evidence relating to outcomes for mothers and newborns, including vulnerable groups
2 Evidence on the cost-effectiveness of case load held practice
3 Impact on midwives working within case load held teams
4 Capacity of the workforce to integrate continuity of carer models
5 Experience of student midwives working within case load held teams and their contribution to women's care

## Evidence relating to outcomes for mothers and newborns, including vulnerable groups

Continuity of carer (case load held practice) is a complex intervention which makes evaluation more difficult. The active ingredients may be the setting for community visits, the personal relationships, frequency of appointments, personnel involved or access to services. This model has the potential to impact on health in pregnancy in terms of the uptake of health advice, regular attendance at appointments, practitioners becoming aware of an individual's normal health parameters, and improved attention to detail and monitoring. The Medical Research Council have highlighted some of the difficulties in evaluating complex care interventions, discussing the role of mediators and unexpected care pathways as there may be many components that interact together (Moore et al., 2015).

DOI: 10.4324/9781003051527-3

Satisfaction

Labour and birth outcomes

Pre-term birth and fetal loss

Postnatal care and outcomes

Vulnerable groups

Cost effectiveness

*Figure 3.1* Themes from the evidence considered

The Cochrane review of midwife led continuity models (Sandall et al., 2016) is the most cited source of evidence about outcomes. This systematic review extracted data from 15 randomised controlled trials across four countries, involving over 17,000 mothers and babies. It is notable that only four studies in the Sandall review evaluated continuity of carer, while the other ten studies evaluated team continuity models. This evidence along with other quantitative and qualitative studies is reviewed under themes extracted from the evidence considered (Figure 3.1).

### *Satisfaction*

Results from the COSMOS (COmparing Standard Maternity care with One-to-one midwifery Support) randomised controlled trial (RCT) (Forster et al., 2016) found that case loading was associated with higher ratings of satisfaction in the antenatal period. Some notable findings were that more women in the case loading group felt they had an active say about decisions regarding their care in pregnancy, that their anxieties and concerns were taken seriously, and midwives seemed less rushed. This was a large Australian study in which 1,156 women at low risk of complications were randomised to case loading care and 1,158 to standard care. A qualitative study by Jepsen et al. (2017) found that partners also welcomed the case loading model as it helped them to feel involved and to develop trust and confidence in the midwife.

Perriman et al. (2018) explored the relational aspect of continuity of carer along with personalised care and the development of trust. These factors may explain the greater satisfaction noted in the COSMOS study, which extends beyond the antenatal period into intrapartum and postnatal periods as well. The strong advocacy element within the case load model is explored by Finlay et al. (2009) and they give several examples where midwives have provided personalised care. One respondent summarised their responsibility and accountability by saying 'people aren't just a faceless person that you are never going to see again' (Finlay et al., 2009, p. 1232). This is echoed by Rayment-Jones et al. (2020) as they describe midwives helping women navigate through the system, enabling early referrals and comprehensive follow up.

### Labour and birth outcomes

McLachlan et al. (2012) found that the epidural rate was significantly lower in women in the case load group than those having standard care (30.5% versus 34.6%; RR 0.88). The Sandall meta-analysis combined results from 14 high quality RCTs and found that 15% fewer women had an epidural, an estimated fall from 270 per 1000 to 229 per 1000 women (Sandall et al., 2016). It is important to note that women with existing serious medical and obstetric complications were not included in this review. The reduction in epidural rate may be due to having a known midwife in labour, a different philosophy of care and more use of community settings for birth. The reduction in epidural rate may impact on the type of birth experienced by women in a case load held team.

Research evidence has highlighted that women with epidurals are more likely to go on to have a ventouse or forceps assisted birth (Newnham et al., 2020). In the Sandall review, rates of spontaneous vaginal birth were higher (relative risk 1.05) and women were also more likely to have an intact perineum in the continuity of carer group (relative risk 1.04). In line with this, fewer women had caesarean births (relative risk 0.92) or instrumental vaginal births (relative risk 0.90). It is important to note that the trials included in the Sandall et al. (2016) review did not include home birth, only four trials included midwifery-led units, and none were exclusively in high-risk populations. This indicates that further research is needed in different settings to evaluate the effectiveness of this model of care.

The labour experience was studied by Gidaszewski et al. (2019) who concluded that the case loading group had reduced interventions in labour, such as amniotomy (35% vs. 50%, OR 0.56) and episiotomy (23% vs. 40%, OR 0.43). There was greater use of water immersion (54% vs. 22%, OR 4.18) and physiological 3rd stage (7% vs. 1%, OR 11.71) indicating that the birth experience can be different in women who are case loaded. This study was a retrospective cohort study of 1000 nulliparous women so lacks an experimental design and the rigour of randomisation.

### Preterm birth and fetal loss

Eight studies in the Sandall et al. (2016) review examined the risk of preterm birth and found a risk reduction of 24% for this outcome. This corresponds with an estimated reduction from 63 preterm births per 1000 to 48 per 1000. Risk of bias was low in these studies indicating that this is high quality evidence. A subsequent study by Turienzo et al. (2016) also found that women randomised to continuity models had a reduced risk of preterm birth. They theorised that women being cared for by known midwives may be more likely to accept help from psychiatric services, be more willing to talk about lifestyle choices such as smoking, and that midwives may be able to recognise problems early and initiate fast access to secondary care. A further RCT exclusively in women with high risk of preterm birth is currently underway, named the POPPIE trial (Pilot study Of midwifery Practice in Preterm birth Including women's Experiences) (Turienzo et al., 2019) where one group has continuity of carer and the other standard care as per usual practice.

*Table 3.1* Activity 3.1 Exploration of preterm births and fetal loss

| *List the known risk factors for Preterm Birth* | *List the known risk factors for fetal loss and/ or neonatal death* |
|---|---|
| Speculate on which of the above could be affected by a Continuity model of care and the process this may follow | Speculate on which of the above could be affected by a Continuity model of care and the process this may follow |
| List evidence you have used to inform your argument | List evidence you have used to inform your argument |

The risk of fetal loss in pregnancy and within one month after birth was also found to be significantly lower (p = 0.04) in the Sandall review by 16%, equating to an estimated risk of 48 per 1000 births reduced from 63 per 1000 births (Sandall et al., 2016). There is insufficient detail in the trials to speculate on why these losses occurred less frequently in the women who received case-loading care. It is a useful exercise to consider which differences in a case-loading model may contribute to benefits in terms of preterm birth and survival.

Use the activity above (Table 3.1) to link your current knowledge base to potential pathways considering the benefits and limitations of pre-term birth and fetal loss.

The reduced risk of neonatal death within one month of birth is an area which needs further exploration. Prematurity, low birth weight and congenital abnormalities account for a high proportion of neonatal deaths. Other risk factors such as smoking, socio economic status, ethnicity and maternal obesity have also been identified as contributing to neonatal death. The mechanism of action for continuity of carer models is unclear however, a complex intervention such as continuity of carer may have a number of active ingredients contributing to these differences and is worthy of debate. Other neonatal outcomes were considered to be secondary outcomes in the Sandall et al. (2016) review. No differences were noted in the proportion of low birthweight infants, apgar score <7 at 5 mins, neonatal convulsions, admission to neonatal unit or length of stay. There were also no differences seen in breastfeeding initiation in the case-loading groups.

**Box 3.1 Activity 3.2**

Reflect on your experiences to date and consider why there are no differences seen in breast feeding initiation. How could you encourage uptake of breast feeding?

*Postnatal care and outcomes*

Few studies have investigated longer term outcomes related to continuity of carer and outcomes relating to postnatal care. Maternal self-confidence, ability to manage motherhood and mental health are all areas that could be explored in future research.

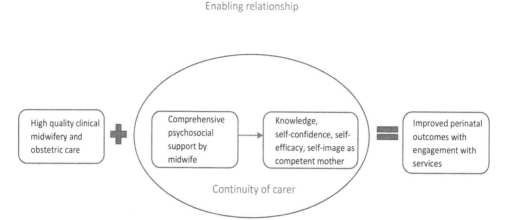

*Figure 3.2* Adapted model by Kemp et al. (2013) to reflect midwifery

The duration of breastfeeding, perineal pain and infection rates have also received little attention in the literature. D'haenens et al. (2019) conducted a systematic review of ten studies comprising two RCTs and eight observational studies. This review looked specifically at the impact of continuity of carer models on physical and mental health within the postnatal period. One limitation of this review is that it included three different concepts of continuity, only one of which was a relational concept which we know as continuity of carer. Most of the studies showed no significant differences in mental health outcomes, however Kemp et al. (2013) found that women were more able to cope with their baby and care for themselves and their baby on the continuity of carer pathway.

Kemp et al. (2013) proposes that improved relationships and engagement with services can lead to improved perinatal outcomes. They propose that the mechanism is via improved knowledge, self-confidence, and competency of the mother as well as obstetric and midwifery care. This is illustrated in Figure 3.2 above.

Perriman et al. (2018) highlight the importance of the interpersonal relationship that develops between women and their case-loading midwife. Person-centred care and empowerment were key concepts emerging from this systematic review and meta-synthesis. Feelings of empowerment and being able to take the lead in decision-making may contribute to the satisfaction with postnatal care and adjustment to motherhood seen in studies by Williams et al. (2010) and Forster et al. (2016).

### *Vulnerable groups*

The potential for women and families to benefit from services can be related to their social environment and their risk of complications. Inequalities are seen in maternal outcomes according to ethnicity and socio economic group (Knight et al., 2019), and therefore it is vital that there is exploration of the benefits of case load held practices in these populations. The NHS Long Term Plan states that services should be targeting midwifery continuity of carer to those women who will benefit most, including those with complex needs (NHS England, 2019). Women who lead more socially complex lives may find it more difficult to engage with services. Measures that improve access and utilisation of services have the potential to improve health and wellbeing outcomes. Homer et al. (2017) highlighted this issue when evaluating care provided at the Albany Midwifery Practice. They analysed data from a 12.5-year period and 57% of the 2568 women were from Black, Asian, and Ethnic minority backgrounds. The setting was Peckham, East London, which is recognised as being an area of socio-economic disadvantage. Positive outcomes were noted in terms of rates of homebirth (43.5%), spontaneous vaginal birth (79.8%) and initiation of breastfeeding (91.5%). An independent evaluation found that compared to other midwifery group practices locally, the Albany Midwifery Practice had a higher homebirth rate, vaginal birth rate, and lower caesarean section rate (Sandall et al., 2001). Levels of continuity of carer were very high as 89% of women were attended in labour by their primary midwife and 98% had an Albany midwife at the birth. Satisfaction and positive experiences were noted in qualitative studies of women's experiences (Huber et al., 2009; Leap et al., 2010).

Rayment-Jones et al. (2015) collected observational data from records of 194 women with complex social factors who presented for maternity care between May 2012 and June 2013. More women in the case load group were referred for multi-disciplinary support services such as psychiatry (56% vs 19%) and domestic violence advocacy (42% vs 18%). Women in the case loading group had fewer antenatal admissions, epidurals in labour, caesarean sections, and neonatal admissions. Non-random allocation and the opportunity for bias in this study limits the strength of this evidence. This study demonstrates the potential mechanisms for improved outcomes in that the case loading group accessed more support services which can contribute to health in pregnancy. Studies documenting the maternity experience of refugees were reviewed by Pangas et al. (2019). They highlighted that continuity with health professionals is important in building trust, communication and reducing inequalities in accessing services.

Women with pre-existing mental health challenges may find benefits in being case loaded. This was highlighted by Hildingsson et al. (2019) who studied women who had been referred to counselling for fear of birth during pregnancy. Having a known midwife during labour and birth had a positive impact on their experience and perception of pain but no difference in the type of birth. Fenwick et al. (2018) raises the point that counselling is more easily implemented in case load models and this way of working has the opportunity to promote mental and social wellbeing. They refer to case load models as an 'untapped resource' to support mental health. A similar view was held by respondents in the Styles et al. (2020) who felt that women with mental illness or a previous traumatic birth should be prioritised for case load held practices, stating that:

> obviously it's always beneficial to everyone, but especially for those women ... [with] social issues, mental health, sexual abuse.... They're not explaining that to everyone they meet, and they're not having to keep going over their story.
>
> (Styles et al., 2020, p. 348)

This finding was also noted in the meta-synthesis of qualitative research by Megnin-Viggars et al. (2015). They identified that the disclosure of negative emotions was most likely to occur if the midwife relationship was continuous throughout pregnancy.

A further area of study has been case-loading in pregnant adolescents, as it is deemed that this cohort are more likely to come from socially disadvantaged backgrounds. Related factors such as low income, housing, social isolation, diet, alcohol use and smoking are described by Allen et al. (2015). A retrospective cohort study based upon records suggests that young women who are case loaded are less likely to have a preterm birth or have babies admitted to neonatal unit, while rates of low birth weight infants and breastfeeding initiation were similar (Allen et al., 2015). Further research is needed in this area as these results are limited by the design of the study, cross over between groups and differences in demographics between the groups studied (Dahlen, 2016). The population were all different but the allocation to groups was not undertaken systematically. One point of note is that authors highlight that more women in the case loading group disclosed mental health problems (24% vs 16%) and illicit drug use (33% vs 24%) to the case loading midwives more than the standard care group. This increased disclosure is an opportunity for further referral and could modify the risk to the pregnancy and fetus. Rayment-Jones et al. (2020) highlight other potential mechanisms of action in women with complex social backgrounds. They report that case loading midwives are more able to engage with women who have barriers to attending appointments due to social factors such as travel, finance, and caring responsibilities.

It is important to note that the Sandall et al. (2016) systematic review did not report on whether outcomes differed for socially disadvantaged women. They recommend that future research should be done in this population and also to determine the mechanisms underpinning any improved outcomes. Rayment-Jones et al. (2020) consider that continuity of carer is not a panacea, as some women may distrust services and be reluctant to accept help with social problems.

## Evidence on the cost-effectiveness of case load held practice

Findings of the Toohill et al. (2012) study suggest that continuity of carer is associated with better outcomes and is less costly than standard care in low risk women. In this non-randomised trial, 52 women received care by the Midwifery Group Practice and 50 received standard care. Positive outcomes were noted in women receiving Midwifery Group Practice care and this model was associated with lower costs from both a hospital and government perspective. This study is limited by its non-randomised design and opportunity for selection bias. Donnellan Fernandez (2013) studied women at moderate obstetric risk who had received Midwifery Group Practice care or standard hospital care in Adelaide during 2004–2010. Women having care under the Midwifery Group Practice had lower rates of induction, epidural, instrumental birth and elective caesarean section. Cost reductions were noted in terms of maternal and neonatal hospitalisation rates and length of stay. It is proposed that continuity models are more efficient as midwives are working flexibly to meet women's needs rather than staffing an institution and waiting for women to come in to the unit (Newton et al., 2019).

Cost outcomes were considered alongside clinical outcomes in the large RCT of 'all risk' women by Tracy et al. (2013). One thousand, seven hundred and thirty-eight women were randomly assigned to case load care or standard care. Costs of all care were calculated, including length of stay, procedures, laboratory tests, imaging and pharmacy. The median difference in cost was Australian $566 less per woman who was cared for under a case load model. Savings were made up of small differences in a number of clinical outcomes such as fewer antenatal appointments, lower rates of assisted birth induction, post partum haemorrhage, and reduced length of postnatal stay. Neonatal outcomes did not differ in this study so no cost savings were realised for neonatal care.

Cost of care for women with complex pregnancies was reviewed by Donnellan Fernandez et al. (2018). This structured review of the literature included three systematic reviews, four RCTs with economic evaluation and two quasi experimental cost studies. The costs varied widely according to funding models and workforce arrangements. The authors found limited evidence to support the cost effectiveness of continuity models for women with complex pregnancies.

## Summary of evidence

The evidence underpinning case load midwifery has been scrutinised and has considered the outcomes measures for mothers and babies that are potentially modified by case load held practice. A vast array of outcomes are described, including the impact on preterm birth, neonatal loss, birth experience, intervention rates and postnatal wellbeing. A consideration of the populations who have increased capacity to benefit from continuity of carer has been presented, such as those from low socioeconomic groups, adolescent mothers, and those with pre-existing mental health conditions. New evidence is emerging in other groups such as women planning a vaginal birth after caesarean (Keedle et al., 2020) and in women with obesity (Denison et al., 2017). The evidence is not clear about the components of the case loading model that are most effective in bringing about these positive outcomes, nor the ways of organising continuity teams or case loading staff.

The evidence points to improved cost-effectiveness for continuity of carer models in women with low to moderate risk of obstetric complications. Further research is needed in women with complex pregnancies. There is also a need to estimate the long-term cost savings associated with the reduction in preterm birth. It is recommended that economic evaluations are built into future studies of case load held practice (Donnellan Fernandez et al., 2019).

## Impact on midwives working within case load held teams

The NHS People Plan discusses working differently to meet client needs while looking after the health and wellbeing of staff (NHS Employers, 2020). This section explores the potential impact on midwives of moving to a case load model from a traditional model of care delivery. Staff retention is a large concern for midwifery employers and midwifery can be a demanding job. This makes it even more important that models of working are good for both the women and midwives working in this role.

### *Negative factors*

Hunter et al. (2019) conducted an online survey of UK midwives in 2017. Of the 1997 respondents, over one third of them scored in the moderate/severe/extreme range for anxiety, depression, and stress. 83% scored moderate or above for personal burnout. This study is limited in that subjects were self-selected, although it does highlight that many midwives are affected by stress, which impacts on their health. Emotional exhaustion is a key component of burnout, and the creation of healthy working conditions is essential in preventing this (Seidler et al., 2014). One of the triggers of burnout is the 'giving of self' nature of work and emotional demands. Several authors have expressed concern that case loading midwives are more at risk of burnout (Sandall, 1997; Newton et al., 2014; Stoll et al., 2019). The study by Stoll et al. (2019) was conducted in Western Canada where midwives exclusively follow a case load held practice. They experienced high levels of burnout which had a negative impact on their personal lives. One in three had seriously considered leaving the profession due to occupational stressors linked to working practices. Midwives in the phenomenological study by Bradfield et al. (2019) also spoke of the personal cost of case loading in terms of sleep, exhaustion, and family time. There can be a blurring of work time and personal time, and on-call duties can be psychologically difficult (Newton et al., 2019).

Young et al. (2015) conducted a phenomenological study of 12 case loading midwives who had experienced burnout. This in-depth exploration exposes the pain of burnout, and dissociation with usual professional values as described here:

> The mobile phone going all the time.... I hated it, I hated the women, I hated midwifery ... that was very frightening, finding myself hating to be a midwife when I have always been exceedingly proud that I was a midwife.
>
> (Young, 2015, p. 205)

Midwifery case loading calls for a high level of commitment and has unpredictable demands. The experience of case loading is not lived by the midwife alone as, as one respondent highlighted the impact on their family:

> When the midwife is on call the whole family is on call, and when she is finally home the family has to be shut down so she can sleep.
>
> (Young, 2015, p. 212)

The issues of work-life balance, sustainability and burnout are also addressed in the thesis by Pace (2018). While there is potential for burnout in the case loading model, several protective factors have also been identified.

### Positive factors

The close relationships that case loading midwives develop with women is thought to add to satisfaction and fulfilment in the role (Sandall, 1997). This was also found by Bradfield et al. (2019) as they acknowledged the personal investment of being 'with woman' and the connections that they felt. Occupational autonomy and flexible working patterns are other positive aspects of working in this way. Balancing home and work life are important in sustaining these models and a working schedule can be managed flexibly to meet both the needs of the woman and the midwife. This can be a challenge at times as noted by a respondent in the Menke et al. (2014) study:

When I first started in Midwifery Group Practice I had the best work life balance, I exercised ... I wasn't totally consumed by the job. My house was always clean. I had really good ability to be able to separate my life. Now though I am totally lost in Midwifery Group Practice.

(Menke et al., 2014, p. 1100)

Several studies have suggested that case loading can have a protective effect against burnout, and that rates are lower than for midwives working in the traditional model. A selection of these studies is summarised in Table 3.2. Studies are limited in that the midwives will have self-selected to work in case load models and may not be representative of all midwives working or yet to work in this role. In addition to this, some studies are hampered by low response rates which may introduce bias in the findings.

Despite the limitations of the study designs and methodology, there seems to be clear evidence that case load held practices can bring about benefits for midwives who choose to work in this way. It is not clear whether this would be the same for all midwives, and the additional commitment of on-call duties may be unmanageable for some midwives and their families. This could lead to work related stress, sickness and attrition, which is something providers are keen to guard against. Some studies have investigated strategies that protect against burnout, so these can be promoted and maintained. Autonomy in working practice, social support and the ability to develop meaningful relationships have been found to be factors that sustain midwives and help to protect against burnout (Sandall, 1997; Collins et al., 2010; Yoshida et al., 2013). Newton et al. (2014) suggests that the personal characteristics and attitudes of some midwives may mean they are drawn to case load practice, and that this strong motivation will influence their success. In their scoping literature review, Sidhu et al. (2020) have summarised the main learning points regarding reducing burnout in midwifery practice. Reflect on your experiences to date in relation to Sidhu et al.'s (2020) main learning points.

*Table 3.2* Studies of burnout related to model of care

| | | |
|---|---|---|
| Ingrid Jepsen et al. (2017) Denmark | Cross sectional survey of 50 midwives | Case load held midwifery was associated with lower burnout scores |
| Dawson et al. (2018) Australia | Cross sectional survey of 542 midwives | Case load held midwives had more positive attitude towards their professional role and lower burnout scores for the work related and personal subscales on burnout inventory |
| Dixon et al. (2017) New Zealand | Cross sectional survey of 1073 midwives | Case load midwives who were self-employed had less burnout and better emotional health than midwives working in an employed capacity. Lower levels of autonomy, professional recognition and empowerment were experienced by the employed midwives |
| Sidhu et al. (2020) | Scoping literature review | Twenty-seven research papers were included in this scoping review. Midwives working in case loading models had significantly lower burnout rates compared with midwives in other models |
| Suleiman-Martos et al. (2020) | Systematic review and meta-analysis | Six studies separating effects of case load working were identified. Concluded that case loading presents with lower levels of burnout than traditional models |

**Box 3.2 Activity 3.3**

Consider the environment you are working within and reflect upon:

- Does the environment make you feel safe and is self-care valued?
- What evidence have you that demonstrates the presence of a supportive manager?
- Is there evidence of on-going continued professional development and education to support you?
- Are there support mechanisms that promote increasing work satisfaction, autonomy and professional relationships?
- Does the organisation promote a family friendly work environment?
- How do staff primarily achieve a work life balance?
- How are staff supported following traumatic experiences?
- What does a healthy work environment look like from your experiences?
- From your experiences, do midwives feel valued?
- Are services being reconfigured to promote continuity of carer models of care?
- Does the environment address the issues of stress, burnout and promote resilience?

## Capacity of the workforce to integrate continuity of carer models

One of the key challenges is the scaling up of continuity of carer in a sustainable way (Sandall et al., 2019). The workforce transformation plans are outlined in NHS guidance, and ask Local Maternity Systems to identify opportunities to implement continuity models and remove barriers (NHS England, 2017). These changes may take time to materialise as they involve significant organisational change and a shift in ideology. A further constraining factor is the staffing crisis evident within the maternity system as there are approximately 3,500 full time positions unfilled, many midwives due to retire and concern about fewer midwives joining from the European Union (RCM, 2017). Staffing shortages are evident with the closure of some freestanding birth centres and diversion of women away from obstetric units at times of peak demand (Blotkamp et al., 2019). This context of staffing strain will make it slower and more onerous to implement continuity models. Despite this, approximately 85% of services across England, Scotland and Wales have started on this path of enactment (Blotkamp et al., 2019). Implementation may be through full case load held practice or via team continuity models. Many areas across the UK have started case load practises with selected groups of women, prioritising those with poorest outcomes and therefore greatest capacity to benefit. This focus on inequality is in line with the NHS Long Term Plan (NHS England, 2019).

The majority of midwives surveyed by Hollins Martin et al. (2020) had positive attitude towards continuity of carer philosophies. Some midwives have expressed concern about the organisational change needed to implement case loading on a wide scale, or could not see themselves juggling home and work life within a continuity of carer model of care (Hollins Martin et al., 2020). The authors go on to say that re-organising services is a 'big ask' of midwives and can see that some are reluctant to do so. An online survey of 798 midwives in the UK highlighted that 24% were willing to work in a case loading team that included intrapartum care and 53% were not (Taylor et al., 2018). These figures were higher when continuity of carer was delivered as part of a team (32% willing, 42% not willing). Newton et al. (2021) reported that willingness to work in a case load model increases when staff are given the opportunity to experience this first hand for a trial period. This aims to help staff to understand the personal benefits of working in this way in terms of flexibility, autonomy and relationship building, rather than just the perceived negatives relating to on-call duties. As the sustainability of the model is dependent on being able to staff it adequately, the potential for growth could be constrained by the proportion of midwives willing to work in this way.

The qualitative enquiry by Styles et al. (2020) followed the journey of one midwifery service in Australia as they have upscaled continuity models. Issues such as replacement for annual leave, sick leave, and upskilling of staff to work across the full scope of practice were some of the areas that needed development. This fits with Taylor et al. (2018) who identified that 53% of the midwives surveyed did not have the clinical confidence to work across all settings. Newton et al. (2019) recommend that managers should enable scheduled paid time for the team to come together for support and distribution of workload. They also forsee that midwives will move in and out of case loading models over their career. This understanding will help managers to plan ahead and be more likely to achieve a sustainable model of care.

The experience of midwives at King's College Hospital in London is described by Holland et al. (2018) in relation to the sustainability of the model. Holland et al. highlight that the use of case loading midwives to fill the gaps of staffing on labour ward must be avoided, as this has an impact on midwife wellbeing and could lead to the midwife being absent for a case loading birth the next day. Teamworking and mutual support are also identified as essential elements in successful case loading. Autonomy over workload, respect for time off and management support with a shared vision were other key features which have helped sustain case loading in this setting (Holland et al., 2018). Threats to midwives' wellbeing include poor staffing and high workload, both of which are thought to contribute to midwifery burnout (Cramer et al., 2019).

The role of maternity support workers is evolving, with the development of the competency, education and career framework (Health Education England, 2019a). The configuration of some case load teams already includes a maternity support worker, for example the team at King's College Hospital have a team leader, five midwives and a support worker (Holland et al., 2018). Support workers can develop long term relationships with women that may enhance communication, health promotion, breastfeeding guidance and mental health support. Models have emerged where maternity support workers act as a second health worker at low-risk births, under the direction of the midwife (Taylor et al., 2018). Support workers may have a key role in helping midwives develop continuity of carer (Health Education England, 2019b), although this role has yet to be fully defined and evaluated.

## Experience of student midwives working within case load held teams and their contribution to women's care

### *Student's experience of case-loading*

The continuity of carer experience is important for students as it can increase exposure to autonomy and decision-making, while gaining a greater understanding of women's social factors and family influences. It is also important for developing key skills, as they may work in a continuity model soon after registration. Students who only understand fragmented care models will be unprepared for job roles upon qualifying. One student on the Bachelor of Science Midwifery programme in the UK has commented that the opportunity allowed her to:

> grow in confidence and experience first-hand the bond that can form between women and midwives through continuity.... It felt really nice being able to follow women through their journeys and lay foundations throughout pregnancy to be able to support them during labour and postnatally. While case loading I felt the weight of responsibility and 'like a midwife' for the first time, despite being overseen.
>
> (Personal communication, 2020)

Continuity of carer can provide unique learning opportunities for students, many of whom state that this is the most rewarding experience of their whole midwifery course (Gray et al., 2016). The woman-centred experience facilitated students to 'bring it all together' in a meaningful way. Theory can be interlinked with practice and there is a perception of having more time to spend listening to women (Sidebotham et al., 2019). A qualitative study by Browne et al. (2014) explored the experience of case loading from the perspective of student midwives, midwifery managers and registered midwives. The importance of relationships and woman-centred care was a key theme. Midwives felt that students can gain a better appreciation of normal midwifery, develop sound clinical decision-making skills and experience the full scope of midwifery practice. The experience helped students feel more confident and they felt it enabled them to practise clinical skills. Women who knew them were more willing to let them participate in learning skills. Some challenges were noted for students in terms of arranging childcare, disruption to their family life and managing their academic workload and personal commitments. This area had been previously studied by Rawnson (2011) who found that despite these challenges, students did not want to let the women down and felt a deep sense of responsibility to meet their expectations.

Some programmes impose a mandatory number of follow-through experiences and this has been described as gruelling by some students. They felt the recruitment process was one of the most stressful elements and feared being rejected. Approaching women felt intrusive and awkward. Fulfilling requirements was also difficult if midwives did not contact them for the labour and birth (Gray et al., 2013). Some participants adopted a superficial, surface approach to meet the University requirements whereas others immersed themselves in the experience and achieved deeper learning. Students need to be well-supported in this learning activity to help them make the most of the opportunity (Gray et al., 2016). New case loading graduates in the study by Cummins et al. (2015) reported a great sense of satisfaction and reward from the two-way interaction and building relationships. One midwife said that by seeing a story unfold it made more sense to her, rather than seeing a snapshot alone. On qualifying, some students feel they need to consolidate their learning before joining a continuity of care model (Kuliukas et al., 2021). The experience of clinical placements was the largest influence of career choices on graduation.

*Women's experience of case-loading by students*

A thorough explanation of women's narratives can be found in the PhD thesis by Rawnson (2018), and a few examples of research studies will be presented here. In a study in Norway from 2009–2010 six midwifery students provided continuity of care to 58 women, with one of them attending the birth and the same student providing postnatal care. Qualitative feedback was given via group interviews of both the mothers and fathers. The participants had positive experiences and spoke about the benefits of continuity in terms of reassurance, trust, confidence and feeling empowered (Aune et al., 2012).

A mixed methods evaluation is presented by Browne & Taylor (2014) which took place in Australia from 2009–2011. Three hundred and fifty-four surveys were completed, which represents a 34% response rate. The mean satisfaction score was 8.88 when women were asked to rate their satisfaction from 1 (not at all satisfied) to 10 (extremely satisfied). Over 67% said the experience was better than they expected, and 62% said that having a student providing continuity made a difference. In the qualitative comments, women appreciated the students' efforts to attend appointments and be on call for them. They felt that being paired with a student meant they had extra attention, support, information, and advocacy. This was also evident in the qualitative study by Rawnson (2018) who described this extra special care as a 'win-win' as the needs of both the student and women are fulfilled. Browne & Taylor (2014) highlight that 15 women scored their satisfaction as four or below out of ten. Some said they felt a sense of responsibility as their labour was quick and the student did not reach them in time. Others reported a lack of commitment from the student in terms of reliability or appreciation of the learning experience.

> Our student was unreliable – often late and absent, always apologetic but generally we gave up expecting her to be there when she said she would be.
> I think the program is fine. My issues are specific to the student I had. I don't think she appreciated the learning opportunity she was presented with.
>
> (Browne et al., 2014, p. e113)

The vast majority of respondents in the Jefford et al. (2020) study provided positive responses from women experiencing case loading by students. This online survey had a 50% response rate and included comments from 946 women. Women found comfort in seeing a familiar face, and the student's presence put them at ease and helped them to feel safe. The authors have questioned whether some students had over-stepped the professional boundaries in a few cases. One woman said her student was always available by text, and another described the student as part of the family. This point indicates the need for adequate preparation of students before embarking on case loading.

---

**Box 3.3 Summary of key points**

- Continuity of carer (case loading) is a complex intervention which makes evaluation difficult.
- Many studies have evaluated team continuity models, with fewer looking at case loading only.

- Case loading is associated with higher ratings of satisfaction in the antenatal, intrapartum and postnatal periods.
- Women feel more involved, less rushed and report more personalised care.
- Continuity is associated with less intervention in labour and a higher rate of spontaneous vaginal births.
- Risk of preterm birth and fetal loss is reduced within continuity models. The reason for this is uncertain.
- Birthweight, neonatal condition at birth and breastfeeding initiation are no different in continuity carer.
- Most studies show no difference in mental health outcomes postnatally.
- Continuity improves relationships and engagement with services. It may facilitate the disclosure of harmful health behaviours and mental health concerns.
- Positive outcomes have been noted in women from low socio-economic groups and marginalised women such as those with mental health problems, pregnant adolescents and refugees.
- Cost reductions have been noted in some studies although the evidence is not conclusive, especially in those with complex pregnancies.
- A large number of midwives are affected by stress, anxiety and depression.
- There is a personal cost of case loading in terms of personal time, uncertainty, restricted social opportunities and family commitments.
- Case loading offers some protective factors against burnout in terms of the quality of relationships, autonomy and flexible working patterns.
- Studies of burnout in midwives may be biased due to self-selection for this role. Many studies report that burnout is not increased in midwives who case load.
- Recruitment of midwives and the sustainability of the model may hinder widespread implementation.
- Management issues such as covering for sickness and annual leave, allowing midwives to rotate out of the model and upskilling should be considered.
- Case loading provides unique learning opportunities for students but can put a burden on them if they have strict requirements to fulfil.
- Women attach great value to student midwives case loading them and report high levels of satisfaction.

## References

Allen, J., Gibbons, K., Beckmann, M., et al. (2015). Does model of maternity care make a difference to birth outcomes for young women? A retrospective cohort study. *International Journal of Nursing Studies*, 52(8): 1332–1342.

Aune, I., Dahlberg, U., & Ingebrigtsen, O. (2012). Parents' experiences of midwifery students providing continuity of care. *Midwifery*, 28(4): 432–438.

Blotkamp, A., Aughey, H., Carroll, F., et al. (2019). *National Maternity and Perinatal Audit: Organisational Report 2019*.

Bradfield, Z., Hauck, Y., Kelly, M., et al. (2019). 'It's what midwifery is all about': Western Australian midwives' experiences of being 'with woman' during labour and birth in the known midwife model. *BMC Pregnancy and Childbirth*, 19(1): 29.

Browne, J., Haora, P.J., Taylor, J., & Davis, D.L. (2014). 'Continuity of care' experiences in midwifery education: Perspectives from diverse stakeholders. *Nurse Education in Practice*, 14(5): 573–578.

Browne, J., & Taylor, J. (2014). 'It's a good thing…': Women's views on their continuity experiences with midwifery students from one Australian region. *Midwifery*, 30(3): e108–e114.

Collins, C., Fereday, J., Pincombe, J., Oster, C., & Turnbull D. (2010). An evaluation of the satisfaction of midwives working in midwifery group practice. *Midwifery*, 26(4): 435–441.

Cramer, E., & Hunter, B. (2019). Relationships between working conditions and emotional wellbeing in midwives. *Women and Birth*, 32(6): 521–532.

Cummins, A., Denney-Wilson, E., & Homer, C. (2015). The experiences of new graduate midwives working in midwifery continuity of care models in Australia. *Midwifery*, 31: 438–444.

D'haenens, F., Van Rompaey, B., Swinnen, E., et al. (2019). The effects of continuity of care on the health of mother and child in the postnatal period: A systematic review. *European Journal of Public Health*, 30(4): 749–760.

Dahlen, H.G. (2016). Continuity of midwifery care models improve outcomes for young women and babies. *Evidence-based nursing*, 19(3): 72–72.

Dawson, K., Newton, M., Forster, D., & McLachlan, H. (2018). Comparing case load and non-case load midwives' burnout levels and professional attitudes: A national, cross-sectional survey of Australian midwives working in the public maternity system. *Midwifery*, 63: 60–67.

Denison, F.C., MacGregor, H., Stirrat, L.I., et al. (2017). Does attendance at a specialist antenatal clinic improve clinical outcomes in women with class III obesity compared with standard care? A retrospective case-note analysis. *BMJ Open*, 7(5).

Dixon, L., Guilliland, K., Pallant, J., et al. (2017). The emotional wellbeing of New Zealand midwives: Comparing responses for midwives in case loading and shift work settings. *New Zealand College of Midwives Journal* (53).

Donnellan Fernandez, R. (2013). Midwifery group practice v standard hospital care: A cost and resource study. Available at: https://dspace2.flinders.edu.au/xmlui/handle/2328/35035 [accessed: 29 December, 2020].

Donnellan Fernandez, R., Creedy, D.K., & Callander, E.J. (2018). Cost-effectiveness of continuity of midwifery care for women with complex pregnancy: A structured review of the literature. *Health Economics Review*, 8(1): 32.

Donnellan Fernandez, R., Scarf, V., Devane, D., et al. (2019). Is midwifery continuity of care cost effective? In C.S. Homer, N. Leap, P. Briodie, & J. Sandall (Eds.), *Midwifery Continuity for Care*. Elsevier.

Fenwick, J., Toohill, J., Slavin, V., et al. (2018). Improving psychoeducation for women fearful of childbirth: Evaluation of a research translation project. *Women and Birth*, 31(1): 1–9.

Finlay, S., & Sandall, J. (2009). 'Someone's rooting for you': Continuity, advocacy and street-level bureaucracy in UK maternal healthcare. *Social Science & Medicine*, 6(8): 1228–1235.

Forster, D., McLachlan, H., Davey, M., Biro, M., Farrell, T., Gold, L., Flood, M., Shafiei, T., & Waldenström, U. (2016). Continuity of care by a primary midwife (case load midwifery) increases women's satisfaction with antenatal, intrapartum and postpartum care: Results from the COSMOS randomised controlled trial. *BMC Pregnancy and Childbirth*, 16(1): 28.

Gidaszewski, B., Khajehei, M., Gibbs, E., et al. (2019). Comparison of the effect of case load midwifery program and standard midwifery-led care on primiparous birth outcomes: A retrospective cohort matching study. *Midwifery*, 69: 10–16.

Gray, J., Leap, N., Sheehy, A., & Homer, C. (2013). Students' perceptions of the follow-through experience in three year bachelor of midwifery programme in Australia. *Midwifery*, 2(4): 400–406.

Gray, J., Taylor, J., & Newton, M. (2016). Embedding continuity of care experiences: An innovation in midwifery education. *Midwifery*, 33: 40–42.

Health Education England (2019a). Maternity support worker competency, education and career development framework. Available at: www.hee.nhs.uk/our-work/maternity/maternity-support-workers [accessed: 30 November, 2020].

Health Education England (2019b). Maternity workforce strategy – Transforming the maternity workforce. Available at: www.hee.nhs.uk/sites/default/files/document/MWS_Report_Web.pdf [accessed: 30 November, 2020].

Hildingsson, I., Rubertsson, C., Karlström, A., et al. (2019). A known midwife can make a difference for women with fear of childbirth-birth outcome and women's experiences of intrapartum care. *Sexual & Reproductive Healthcare*, 21: 33–38.

Holland, S., & Wiseman, O. (2018). Is case loading sustainable? Lessons from the front line at King's College Hospital. *Practising Midwife*. Available at: www.all4maternity.com/is-caseloading-sustainable-lessons-from-the-front-line-at-kings-college-hospital/ [accessed: 30 November, 2020]

Hollins Martin, C., MacArthur, J., Martin, C., et al. (2020). Midwives' views of changing to a Continuity of Midwifery Care (CMC) model in Scotland: A baseline survey. *Women and Birth: Journal of the Australian College of Midwives*, 33: e409–e419.

Homer, C.S., Leap, N., Edwards, N., et al. (2017). Midwifery continuity of carer in an area of high socio-economic disadvantage in London: A retrospective analysis of Albany Midwifery Practice outcomes using routine data (1997–2009). *Midwifery*, 48: 1–10.

Huber, U.S., & Sandall, J. (2009). A qualitative exploration of the creation of calm in a continuity of carer model of maternity care in London. *Midwifery*, 25(6): 613–621.

Hunter, B., Fenwick, J., Sidebotham, M., & Henley, J. (2019). Midwives in the united kingdom: Levels of burnout, depression, anxiety and stress and associated predictors. *Midwifery* 79: 102526.

Jefford, E., Nolan, S.J., Sansone, H., et al. (2020). 'A match made in midwifery': Women's perceptions of student midwife partnerships. *Women and Birth*, 33(2): 193–198.

Jepsen, I., Mark, E., Foureur, M., et al. (2017). A qualitative study of how case load midwifery is experienced by couples in Denmark. *Women and Birth*, 30(1): e61–e69.

Keedle, H., Peters, L., Schmied, V., et al. (2020). Women's experiences of planning a vaginal birth after caesarean in different models of maternity care in Australia. *BMC Pregnancy and Childbirth*, 20(1): 1–15.

Kemp, L., Harris, E., McMahon, C., et al. (2013). Benefits of psychosocial intervention and continuity of care by child and family health nurses in the pre-and postnatal period: Process evaluation. *Journal of Advanced Nursing*, 69(8): 1850–1861.

Knight H., Bunch K., & Tuffnell D. (2019). Saving lives, improving mothers' care. Lessons learned to inform maternity care from the UK and Ireland Confidential Enquiries into Maternal Deaths and Morbidity 2015–17. Available at: www.npeu.ox.ac.uk [accessed: 7 September, 2020].

Kuliukas, L., Bayes, S., Geraghty, S., et al. (2021). Graduating midwifery students' preferred model of practice and first job decisions: A qualitative study. *Women and Birth*, 34(1): 61–68.

Leap, N., Sandall, J., Buckland, S., et al. (2010). Journey to confidence: Women's experiences of pain in labour and relational continuity of care. *Journal of Midwifery & Women's Health*, 55(3): 234–242.

McLachlan, H.L., Forster, D.A., Davey, M.-A., et al. (2012). Effects of continuity of care by a primary midwife (case load midwifery) on caesarean section rates in women of low obstetric risk: The COSMOS randomised controlled trial. *BJOG: An International Journal of Obstetrics & Gynaecology*, 119(12): 1483–1492.

Megnin-Viggars, O., Symington, I., Howard, L.M., et al. (2015). Experience of care for mental health problems in the antenatal or postnatal period for women in the UK: A systematic review and meta-synthesis of qualitative research. *Archives of Women's Mental Health*, 18(6): 745–759.

Menke, J., Fenwick, J., Gamble, J., et al. (2014). Midwives' perceptions of organisational structures and processes influencing their ability to provide case load care to socially disadvantaged and vulnerable women. *Midwifery*, 30(10): 1096–1103.

Moore, G.F., Audrey, S., Barker, M., et al. (2015). Process evaluation of complex interventions: Medical Research Council guidance. *British Medical Journal*, 350.

Newnham, E.C., Moran, P.S., Begley, C.M., et al. (2020). Comparison of labour and birth out-comes between nulliparous women who used epidural analgesia in labour and those who did not: A prospective cohort study. *Women and Birth*. https://doi.org/10.1016/j.wombi.2020.09.001

Newton, M.S., Dawson, K., Forster, D., et al. (2021). Midwives' views of case load midwifery – comparing the case load and non-case load midwives' opinions. A cross-sectional survey of Australian midwives. *Women and Birth*, 34(1): e47–e56.

Newton, M.S., White, J., & Briodie, P. (2019). How can managers make midwifery continuity of care work? In H.C.N. Leap, P.M. Brodie, & J. Sandell (Eds.), *Midwifery Continuity of Care*, 2nd ed. Elsevier.

Newton, M., McLachlan, H., Willis, K., & Forster, D. (2014). Comparing satisfaction and burnout between case load and standard care midwives: Findings from two cross-sectional surveys conducted in Victoria, Australia. *BMC Pregnancy and Childbirth*, 14(1).

NHS Employers (2020). We are the NHS: People Plan 2020/21 action for us all. NHS Improvement. Available at: www.england.nhs.uk/publication/we-are-the-nhs-people-plan-for-2020-21-action-for-us-all/ [accessed: 30 December, 2020].

NHS England (2017). Implementing better births: Continuity of carer. Available at www.england.nhs.uk/publication/implementingbetter-births-continuity-of-carer [accessed: 29 November, 2020].

NHS England (2019). NHS Long Term Plan: Online version of the NHS Long Term Plan. London: NHS England. Available at: www.longtermplan.nhs.uk/online-version/ [accessed: 29 November, 2020].

Pace, C.A. (2018). *Co-creation of Guiding Principles and a Practical Framework for a Midwifery Continuity of Carer Model: A Cooperative Inquiry with Midwives*. Robert Gordon University [online], MRes thesis. Available at: https://openair.rgu.ac.uk [accessed: 30 December, 2020].

Pangas, J., Ogunsiji, O., Elmir, R., et al. (2019). Refugee women's experiences negotiating motherhood and maternity care in a new country: A meta-ethnographic review. *International Journal Of Nursing Studies*, 90: 31–45.

Perriman, N., Davis, D.L., & Ferguson, S. (2018). What women value in the midwifery continuity of care model: A systematic review with meta-synthesis. *Midwifery*, 62: 220–229.

Rawnson, S. (2011). A qualitative study exploring student midwives' experiences of carrying a case load as part of their midwifery education in England. *Midwifery*, 27(6): 786–792.

Rawnson, S. (2018). *Stories of Companionship and Trust: Women's Narratives of their Student Midwife Case Loading Experience*. Bournemouth: Bournemouth University.

Rayment-Jones, H., Murrells, T., & Sandall, J. (2015). An investigation of the relationship between the case load model of midwifery for socially disadvantaged women and childbirth outcomes using routine data: A retrospective, observational study. *Midwifery*, 31(4): 409–417.

Rayment-Jones, H., Silverio, S.A., Harris, J., et al. (2020). Project 20: Midwives' insight into continuity of care models for women with social risk factors: What works, for whom, in what circumstances, and how. *Midwifery*, 84: 102654.

Royal College of Midwives (2017). The gathering storm: England's midwifery workforce challenges. Available at: www.rcm.org.uk/media/2374/the-gathering-storm-england-s-midwifery-workforce-challenges.pdf [accessed: 19 February, 2019].

Sandall J, Soltani H, Shennan A, et al. (2019). Implementing midwife-led continuity models of care and what do we still need to find out? Available at: www.evidentlycochrane.net/midwife-led-continuity-of-care/ [accessed: 9 September, 2020].

Sandall, J. (1997). Midwives' burnout and continuity of care. *British Journal of Midwifery*, 5(2): 106–111.

Sandall, J., Coxon, K., Mackintosh, N., Rayment-Jones, H., Locock, L., & Page, L. (2016). *Relationships: The pathway to safe, high-quality maternity care*. Report from the Sheila Kitzinger symposiumOctober 2015. Green Templeton College, Oxford.

Sandall, J., Davies, J., & Warwick, C. (2001). *Evaluation of the Albany Midwifery Practice (Final Report)*. London: King's College Hospital NHS Trust.

Seidler, A., Thinschmidt, M., Deckert, S., et al. (2014). The role of psychosocial working conditions on burnout and its core component emotional exhaustion: A systematic review. *Journal of Occupational Medicine and Toxicology*, 9(1): 10.

Sidebotham, M., & Fenwick, J., (2019). Midwifery students' experiences of working within a midwifery case load model. *Midwifery*, 74: 21–28.

Sidhu, R., Bowen, S., Shapiro, K., & Stoll, K. (2020). Prevalence of and factors associated with burnout in midwifery: A scoping review. *European Journal of Midwifery*, 4.

Stoll, K., & Gallagher, J. (2019). A survey of burnout and intentions to leave the profession among Western Canadian midwives. *Women and Birth*, 32(4): e441–e449.

Styles, C., Kearney, L., & George, K. (2020). Implementation and upscaling of midwifery continuity of care: The experience of midwives and obstetricians. *Women and Birth*, 33(4): 343–351.

Suleiman-Martos, N., Albendín-García, L., Gómez-Urquiza, J.L., et al. (2020). Prevalence and predictors of burnout in midwives: A systematic review and meta-analysis. *International Journal of Environmental Research and Public Health*, 17(2): 641.

Taylor, B., Cross-Sudworth, F., & McArthur, C. (2018). Better births and continuity: Midwifery survey results. Birmingham: University of Birmingham. Available at: www.birmingham.ac.uk/Documents/college-mds/applied-health/better-birth-and-continuity.pdf [accessed: 28 December, 2020].

Taylor, B., Henshall, C., Goodwin, L., et al. (2018). Task shifting midwifery support workers as the second health worker at a home birth in the UK: A qualitative study. *Midwifery*, 62: 109–115.

Toohill, J., Turkstra, E., Gamble, J., et al. (2012). A non-randomised trial investigating the cost-effectiveness of Midwifery Group Practice compared with standard maternity care arrangements in one Australian hospital. *Midwifery*, 28(6): e874–e879.

Tracy, S.K., Hartz, D.L., Tracy, M.B., Allen, J., Forti, A., Hall, B., et al. (2013). Case load midwifery care versus standard maternity care for women of any risk: M@NGO, a randomised controlled trial. *The Lancet*, 382(9906): 1723–1732.

Turienzo, C., Bick, D., Bollard, M., et al. (2019). POPPIE: Protocol for a randomised controlled pilot trial of continuity of midwifery care for women at increased risk of preterm birth. *Trials*, 20(1): 271.

Turienzo, C., Sandall, J., & Peacock, J. (2016). Models of antenatal care to reduce and prevent preterm birth: A systematic review and meta-analysis. *BMJ Open*, 6(1).

Williams, K., Lago, L., Lainchbury, A., et al. (2010). Mothers' views of case load midwifery and the value of continuity of care at an Australian regional hospital. *Midwifery*, 26(6): 615–621.

Yoshida, Y., & Sandall, J. (2013). Occupational burnout and work factors in community and hospital midwives: A survey analysis. *Midwifery*, 29(8): 921–926.

Young, C.M., Smythe, L., & Couper, J.M. (2015). Burnout: Lessons from the lived experience of case loading midwives. *International Journal of Childbirth*, 5(3): 154–165.

# 4 Practicalities

## Student experiences of case load held practice

*Ellen Kitson-Reynolds and Kate Ashforth*

## Introduction

We have presented the political and professional context of continuity of carer and how systems are set up across the UK compared to other parts of the globe. The evidence base surrounding case-loading and related health benefits have equally been considered alongside the impact on those undertaking this model and approach to care. The previous chapter has started to engage you in considering the evaluation of new service set ups and the auditing or researching of existing services and has evidenced this through a small qualitative study presentation. Well-planned evaluative activities highlight to many interested parties, (i.e., funders, service users, leads in maternity services, national and local monitoring groups) how effective and true to the design services are for all involved, and where there are specific needs to be addressed. So how do you go about setting up a case load or continuity of carer experience that will provide you with the skills as both a student and, more latterly, as a qualified midwife? This chapter aims to provide you with tools for critical consideration and application, linking to you in your current context and your ability to achieve a meaningful continuity of carer experience.

As with many activities within midwifery pre-registration preparation curricula, there are many layers to the events planned and undertaken, such as: passing the module; passing the course; acquiring skills for undertaking the role when qualified; preparation for revalidation; career planning, and the development of a three to five-year plan; preparation for the future workforce, including writing your curriculum vitae and personal statements; linking with practice partner activities as part of the team (PMA, statutory and mandatory training and clinical debriefing, etc); evaluation of 'you' and your values and belief systems; outcomes for women and their families. These 'layers' change meaning to you dependent upon the part of the academic programme you are within i.e., year 1, year 2 and year 3. You will build a more critical and analytical perspective with your evolving knowledge, understanding and experiences that shape the type of practitioner you aspire to become. In year 1 you take more of an observational role whilst starting to reflect upon how the theory applies to the real-world clinical practice setting. By the time you commence your third/final year you will have developed personal leadership skills to manage time and resources appropriately and demonstrate self-management. Similarly, by the mid to end of your final year of training you exude proof that you are an insightful analytical thinker with the ability to problem solve and to generate evidence for the enhancement of practice (NMC, 2019).

DOI: 10.4324/9781003051527-4

As highlighted in previous chapters, midwifery practice is an ever evolving, often challenging profession. Working in partnership with other health and social care professionals and agencies, service users, and families in all settings ensures the clinical decisions you make are informed, shared and owned by all involved. By the time you register as a qualified midwife you will have the skills base to manage your own well-being, for example, professional and personal emotions and stress by following a strength based (Saleebey, 2013) and solution focussed approach (Lewis, 2020), to 'empower and strengthen the capabilities of women' to take responsibility for their own health (NMC, 2019).

This chapter has a practical focus, therefore comprises several questions that you may consider using as checklists. These points for your consideration are available in the final chapter as a resource that you can add to as you feel appropriate, and as fits with your education provider requirements.

## Pre-planning

Activity 4.1 has been designed for you to complete prior to the start of your case load experience and then repeated midway and at the end of your pre-registration programme. It is more effective to complete the answers without referring to previous attempts so that you can compare previous answers and what this means to you in your reality. You can also review this activity at key points through your career and as your personal circumstances change.

### Box 4.1 Activity 4.1

Having read the previous chapters, and prior to starting the planning for your case load experience, list the following:

- What makes me excited about undertaking a continuity of carer/case load experience?
- What am I most anxious about with starting a case load experience?
- What are my external/personal factors and how will these impact on my ability to undertake a case load experience?
- What am I not prepared/able to commit to for a case load experience?
- What are the 'trade offs' to achieve successful case load experiences? (i.e., what am I prepared to change or relinquish to achieve the case load?)
- What do I, as the student midwife, want the woman to gain from me providing continuity of care for them?
- Am I committed to delivering person-centred care?

As you traverse the continuity of carer preparation and delivery, consider what natural strengths you must bring to the profession, thus enhancing the experiences of women and their families. Recalling the values-based enquiry journey in Chapter 1 remind yourself of 'the head' – your academic knowledge and practical skills; 'the heart' – the kindness, care and compassion; and 'the nerve' – the courage you have and your ability to advocate for others. This continuously shapes you to becoming the midwife you dream of becoming. Ask yourself how you are going to incorporate this into your case load journey.

You might be undertaking a continuity of carer case load experience as part of a course module, if so, what are the requirements of the module learning outcomes and your course provider? It may be that you have a pre-requisite number for your case load to be achieved prior to qualification. It may be that the number of women in your case load needed as part of your programme requirements can be spread over a long period of time so do think about how many you wish to achieve by certain points in your training. You would possibly not want to leave them all to the final months of your programme when you have other commitments to achieve, and equally you would not want to complete them all at the start of your programme when the like-lihood of being semi-autonomous and independent in your decision-making and care provision is reduced. Think through what the requirements are for minimum numbers of visits for it to count as continuity of carer, and then consider what you would be happy to provide for it to feel like continuity of carer.

Consider what you want to commit to and what the barriers might be to achieving your potential in the case load. This could be due to your perceived level of confidence, how much time is required, you might have your own childcare to organise and you will have other academic deadlines to factor in. Make sure you scrutinise your programme calendar, including academic submission dates. Devising your own timeline for each year is recommended where you can plot key things not only in the course but events in your personal world to show you where you have space and time to commit to clinical on call work, and where your 'bottle necks' may be that you need to avoid. There is little point in planning a case load where women are due to birth when you are on your annual leave or when your dissertation is due.

You might have the flexibility to choose who you want to be supervised by. It might be that you will have direct supervision by several different midwives. For some students, they want to experience a diverse range of clinical practice delivery and so opt to work across a few teams for their case load. Other students are allocated to a team and for pragmatic reasons they take on a case load while they are there. Consider which midwives you have worked with before and which days they have a clinic and if those days work for you and your academic/university commitments. You may be required to negotiate what you are able/allowed to miss in terms of the rest of the course for the case load and if it is different depending on whether it is antenatal or intrapartum care provision.

## Planning and set up

It takes time to organise your case load, especially if it is the first time you have undertaken it. For many students, they are not fully informed of the complex back-ground activities midwives conduct until they qualify and then are expected to per-form them themselves. Accompany your practice supervisor to see what they do when you are not with them. This way you can start to appreciate the information gathering and preparation, referrals and review of investigation results etc, that happens prior to any contact with the women. As you start to prepare for the case load experience review the questions in table 4.1 as a guide to your thinking. This is meant to encou-rage you to think in relation to your clinical context and not provide you with the answers. This is to facilitate flexibility and individualisation in the care planning with women.

*Table 4.1* Planning and set up questions

| | |
|---|---|
| Paperwork and documentation | • Consider what paperwork you need for booking, antenatal appointments, blood tests, referrals etc and ensure that you have these available to you during the visit. If your Trust has electronic forms of documentation, ensure that you have access and if your practice supervisor is required to be present to log you into any online resources.<br><br>• Think through issues of GDPR (2018). How will you keep records of the interactions you have with women, their families and other multi-professional groups? If travelling between venues, how will you keep anonymised paper records safely so that if, on the rare occasion, you lost them the details of the woman would not be identifiable?<br><br>• How will you update any GP and hospital digital records if required?<br><br>• Does your organisation require you to have all documentation entries countersigned by the responsible practitioner? If so, how will you achieve this? |
| Setting up of case load contract (refer to Chapter 10 for template examples) | Best practice ensures completion of a contract between you, your practice supervisor and the woman.<br><br>• Have you identified and gained agreement to case load with a particular midwife?<br><br>• How will you work together?<br><br>• What are the expectations of you and the practice supervisor?<br><br>• What happens if you are unavailable to attend a planned appointment?<br><br>• When you have identified your case load, who is going to communicate with the woman to ask if she would like you to case load her?<br><br>• How will you devise your contract of commitment with the woman?<br><br>• Does your programme education team/university need to counter sign the contract?<br><br>• Where will this be stored? |
| Yours and your practice supervisor's expectations | • What do you hope to achieve from this case load experience? Consider a mixture of women for your case load experiences i.e. primiparous, multiparous, VBAC, mental health concerns, safeguarding. Sometimes you are not trying to learn complexity/referrals but 'just' the continuity and being with woman so you may wish for a less complex additional care needs scenario.<br><br>• Who do you want to case load (in terms of context, learning experience rather than person)?<br><br>• How many appointments are you expected to attend and how many are reasonable to miss?<br><br>• How will you undertake a tripartite communication? (you, practice supervisor and woman).<br><br>• Think through the requirements of the standards for student supervision and assessment (SSSA) (NMC, 2018) and the level you are at in your training. What are the expectations of you at the level of experience you are at, and how do you interpret 'under direct supervision'? You need to be able to work relatively autonomously at some point during the case load so starting from mid-point of your programme is realistic. While it may be a busy time for you, consider how your practice would be different if you did one or two towards the end of training just when you are about to qualify.<br><br>• How will you demonstrate an ethical understanding of the case load experience and safe professional practice? |

| | |
|---|---|
| What are the women's expectations of you? | • Define your professional boundaries before you start so that you are clear prior to discussion of care planning with the woman. |
| | • It is strongly recommended that you do not use your personal mobile phone for communications with the client(s). You need to agree with your practice supervisor how you will contact the women on your case load and how they will contact you. It may be that your organisation has a work phone that you can use or a work email. If you use this form of digital communication, remember that this is a contemporary record and professional language must be used. It may be that the women contact you via the Trust's contact number and the Trust contact you. |
| | • You need to ensure that the women contact the appropriate departments in the case of a problem as you might not be able to respond to their messages in a timely way. |
| | • How will you ensure collaborative working/shared decision-making? |
| | • If you make an agreed plan you are expected to be reliable and follow through the activity. |
| Planning for the unexpected | • What happens if it goes wrong? Who will you call if you are at a visit on your own and you encounter a problem? |
| | • Who do you report back to? |
| | • What happens if you are not able to attend at short notice – who do you call i.e., duty manager, midwife, women etc? |
| Equipment | • Who in your organisation is responsible for providing students with equipment? |
| | • Who is responsible for ensuring the equipment is in working order and restocked? |
| | • Some organisations have student case load held bags – if so, where are they stored and are they available when you require them? |
| | • Do you have a signing in and out process for borrowing equipment? |
| | • Does the practice supervisor or the midwifery team have spare equipment if you want to do a home visit? |
| Risk assessing | • Who has direct accountability and responsibility for the case load and activity? |
| | • What responsibility does the Trust and university have towards you and have you completed a risk assessment form for the case load experience? Have you got this countersigned by your practice supervisor and/or midwifery academic assessor (NMC, 2018). |
| | • Can you use risk assessment and management strategies to demonstrate adherence to safe practice by ensuring the safety of yourself as a practitioner, your client and others who you case load? |
| Work/life balance | • Have you considered the level of commitment you can provide to the case load at this time in your programme and life circumstances? |
| | • Have you considered and agreed travel arrangements and what happens at different time of the day and night? It may be that you use public transport, so consider availability across the day and week. |
| | • Have you factored in your non-practice obligations and commitments i.e., childcare – school picking up time etc? |

Lone working
- What is the lone working policy of the Trust/university regarding home visits conducted by a lone student?
- Who do you contact to say you are going out to undertake a home visit and what do you do when you have finished the visit?
- Do you have a code word or phrase to alert your practice supervisor if you find yourself in an unsafe or emergency situation?
- Is it a safe time of day to go to the appointment, e.g., is it in daylight, winter or summer for the location?
- Who will you contact if there are any concerns?
- How will you communicate the findings of this visit to the practice supervisor?
- Are there any known safeguarding concerns that could comprise your safety?
- Are visits and communications outside the agreements permissible? Consider why this would be an issue.

Follow up activities
- When referrals need to be made to, for example, consultants, is the practice supervisor in agreement for you to do them and copy them into emails?
- If requesting tests and investigations, it is typically the responsibility of the person requesting to follow up on the results. Who will check and action blood results and other tests/investigations?

Friends and family
- Sometimes you may be approached to case load a friend or member of your family. What are the local guidelines regarding this?
- How does this apply to you as a student?
- Who do you need to gain permissions from?
- How is the role of the PMA used to support this request?

## Undertaking the experience

Remember that this is your case load experience as much as it is for the woman and her family. This means that you are starting to take professional responsibility, albeit under direct supervision, to engage in decision-making processes within a multi professional team and with the woman and her family. As you progress through your training programme you should be assuming greater prowess in thinking through the scenario, risk assessing it, clinically evaluating and considering differential diagnoses and making decisions and action plans for yourself. As you start to develop these clinical skills, you will make errors of judgement. You will forget aspects of care, policy guidance and process. It is normal and ok. You are expected to discuss your critical thinking and clinical reasoning skills with your experienced practice supervisor who will guide you, without telling you, through your thinking processes. Few students appear to worry about being wrong or say that they do not have enough experience of working with midwives who engage them in this skill. As a qualified and experienced midwife, it is not uncommon to talk out loud your clinical reasoning of unusual or complex cases with colleagues. It is a valuable skill that demonstrates safety in patient care. Whilst it is acceptable in your first year of practice to ask your practice supervisor what to do, there will be an expectation for you to start to work autonomously and develop leadership skills to communicate initially using a tool such as an SBAR (ACT Academy, n.d.), then present a plan and engage in a professional discussion as your knowledge and experiences develop. Table 4.2 provides further questions for you to consider, in addition to those in Table 4.1.

*Table 4.2* Questions to consider as you undertake your experience

| | |
|---|---|
| Emotional | • It is not uncommon for women to share very emotional prior birth experiences which may not be part of the planned interaction. If this occurs how will you support her, showing kindness and compassion? How will you be supported in this? |
| Engaging with other health care professionals | • Have you got opportunities to learn with, and from, other healthcare professionals so that you develop competence in interprofessional practice to meet the needs of women and their families requiring maternity services? |
| | • How do you communicate with other professionals and agencies working in collaboration with maternity services, to ensure that the needs of individuals, families and communities are met? |
| Evaluate/reflect on practice | • Are you achieving and doing what you set out to do? |
| | • What work is needed outside of the actual appointments? can you see how this might impact your life as a qualified midwife with a larger case load? |
| | • Are you effectively managing your time and prioritising workloads to sustain efficient and effective practice while demonstrating self-management? |
| | • Consider how your reflective activities will develop your analytical skills to debate, problem solve and make robust clinical care plans to enhance quality care within a changing health and social care environment whilst demonstrating self-management. |
| You and your Practice supervisor | • Is your practice supervisor using guiding hands or controlling hands? |
| | • Are you being supported, and do you feel as though it is your case load? How can this be improved? Are you taking the lead? |
| | • If not, do you feel able to discuss this with your practice supervisor in a professional manner? How might you introduce this conversation? Think about your aims of the conversation, what do you want to change? |
| | • How do women contact you or the midwife between appointments? Does your practice supervisor include you in these conversations? |
| | • Do you feel able to challenge perceived poor practices? |
| Tool kits | • Do you have a support network for you to debrief and to 'catch you if you fall'? |
| | • Have you got notebooks with contacts and for useful info as you go along i.e. telephone numbers for day assessment unit, labour ward, scan dept and how to fill out blood forms or how to request referrals? |

**Box 4.2 Activity 4.2**

You are actively participating as the lead decision maker for a primiparous woman who is 36 weeks' gestation at low risk of complications. She presents to the birth centre with a blood pressure recording of 140/82. You leave her and enter the main office where your practice supervisor is, and you provide a hand over as above. Your practice supervisor asks you for more information than this.

- How would you present this using SBAR (or equivalent)?
- What else do you need to know, are there any other symptoms?
- What diagnosis are you thinking?
- Are there any other differential diagnoses?
- Tell your practice supervisor what you need to do.

a   What was her booking blood pressure?
b   Have you repeated the blood pressure?
c   Do you need to consider a urinalysis and/or bloods?
d   Who do you need to call? E.g. day assessment unit.
e   Think about when this information would be critical.

## Evaluating the experience

After your experience look back at the head, heart and nerve and ask yourself if you are behaving as the midwife you wanted to become. Use a reflective tool such as (Ashforth & Kitson-Reynolds, 2018; Gibbs, 1988; Johns, 2009) to reflect in practice rather than just on practice (Schon, 1991) to demonstrate you are a responsive practitioner. Talking aloud techniques may help with this activity especially within a

- What were the challenges for you throughout your case load experience and consider if they could have been avoided?
- What was the impact on you and your practice supervisor, if any?
- Did you struggle with work/life balance?
- Did the case load give you what you had expected?
- Are you becoming the midwife you wanted to be?
- Will your experience of the student case load influence how you work with students once you are qualified as a practice supervisor?
- Did you enjoy it?
- How do you feel knowing that you are part of the woman's experience?
- How does it make you feel about working in a continuity of carer team as a qualified midwife?
- Do you think it would be achievable?
- Have you developed any strategies to prevent burnout?
- How has your continuity of carer case load experience provided safe care to meet the physical, psychological, environmental, social, emotional and spiritual needs of women within diverse realities?

*Figure 4.1* Questions for reflection

restorative clinical supervision session with a PMA, reflecting with peer groups in an academic setting, reflecting with the practice supervisor, practice assessor or academic assessor (NMC, 2018). It may be that you are required to provide a formal written reflection for your practice assessment document or academic module. It is best practice to reflect as you go along to identify key learning points along the way and show how this has influenced your practice.

As a qualified midwife, receiving feedback from the women is essential to show professional development and revalidation evidence (NMC, 2017). Receiving user feedback is useful to support you with thinking through what can you put into your future practice. Whilst it is delightful to receive positive feedback that people think you are fabulous, consider how you can develop from more meaningful constructive feedback (Figure 4.1). Typically, growth comes with unexpected feedback and feed forward (Brown, 2015).

---

**Box 4.3 Vignette 4.1**

As a student midwife, I had been excited and nervous about starting my case load experience. I loved working in antenatal clinics and wanted to take more responsibility for the women for whom I was providing care, and I wanted them to claim me as 'their midwife'. When Ellen introduced the case load experience to us, she did so alongside mention of a decision-making module based in the academic side of the course, and it was something that I was looking forward to as Ellen was well-known for interesting and interactive lectures. I knew that the case load itself would give me an even greater insight into my own practice and that this would be supported by the decision-making work.

I knew that I wanted to work alongside my community mentor, Jaki, for my case load experience. We had worked together previously, and I admired her practice. Furthermore, we trusted each other: I knew she would push me to be the best version of the midwife I wanted to be and would also shine a spotlight on any areas of my practice that she thought needed it. In turn, she trusted me to escalate concerns to her and to practise within my own capabilities. We had always had excellent lines of communication and so I knew that if I struggled at any point, I would be able to ask her for help without feeling stupid. Despite my excitement, I was also terrified that I would never be able to provide women with the level of care that they deserved, and I worried that I would be good enough for them. This fear has plagued me for most of my adult life, and starting the case load exacerbated it. It did not change until I entered my third year of training and realised that I had the most incredible team of midwives (both clinical and academic) cheering me on and telling me I could do it. At that point I finally realised that if such amazing women were supporting me and rallying around me, then I should trust them. It was a turning point in my training: I relaxed and stopped worrying about whether I was good enough, and I trusted that I was. Do not confuse that trust with complacency, I still worked hard and poured my heart and soul into my training, I continued to reflect and critique my practice, but I laid the inner critic to rest.

When Jaki and I sat down to discuss the case load, I knew that she had very high expectations of me. For her, the case load meant women I would care for, supported by her. She would by no means leave me unsupported, but neither would she see the women for me on a regular basis. I think that was an unspoken understanding that we had: she expected me to be able to manage other deadlines and commitments, and to not let the women's care suffer because of them. I knew that giving some of her own case load to me to care for was a huge sacrifice on her part because her antenatal case load is the part of her job she holds dearest. For her, it is the heart of her midwifery. It is continuity, love, education, support, evidence-based, but also pink and fluffy. She firmly believes that setting women up antenatally with the skills and resources they need enables them to flourish in labour, birth and beyond. As such, when I first started my case load experience, I was desperate to do a good job, not just for myself and the women, but also for Jaki. I wanted to show her everything that I had learned over the course so far, and I wanted her to think I was doing a good job.

For me the initial booking appointment was the most important, it was the 'getting to know you' appointment. Even now, having been qualified for two and a half years, it is the appointment I treasure the most because it gives me and the woman the chance to get to know each other. It sets the scene for our ongoing professional relationship. Jaki expected me to carry these out myself just as much as I wanted to carry them out myself, and I expect the same of students who ask to case load women through my clinic as well. Students who ask to pick up a case load later in pregnancy make me question their commitment to the women, and I wonder whether they have lost sight of the beauty and the essence of the case load experience: to provide holistic woman-centred continuity of carer. Nowhere does it say that continuity from 34 weeks' pregnant to day two postnatal constitutes continuity of carer. By that point, women have claimed their midwife as their own and it is very difficult to forge a meaningful relationship with a woman if they feel as though you have joined the party late, just for convenience. Case loading is about providing continuity of carer for the women as much as they are about providing students with a learning opportunity, they are about making the woman feel valued and important. Similarly, dipping in and out of women's appointments did not sit well with me as a student and I do not accept it from students with whom I work now either. While it is understandable that there are external factors that may preclude attendance at every appointment, the expectation is that the course is preparing you for real world midwifery practice and when you have a case load of women to care for, you must care for them.

For me, timing of case load was important. I undertook my case load of four halfway through my second year, and they all birthed a few months into my third year. At this point I then began a case load of two further women, both of whom birthed just before I completed my studies. There was a marked difference in the level of autonomy I felt between the two sets of case loads': Jaki had much less direct supervision over me during the second set, and I felt as though I was a proper midwife by the time, I discharged the last woman from midwifery care. The sense of achievement I felt upon completing the experience was immense. It was hugely gratifying to know that I had been allowed to follow six women on their journeys to becoming parents, and I had learnt so much about providing care to six very different women with very different expectations and care needs. In addition, I learnt a lot about myself as a person and as a midwife. I saw the midwife I had become, and I could clearly see the values that mattered the most to me: holistic, individualised woman-centred care that made the woman feel loved and supported, all of which was bound in safe, evidence-based practice.

My case load experience was not plain sailing, by any stretch of the imagination. One woman seemed to hate me, and we just did not gel, although she did not ever ask to not see me, and she gave me positive feedback. I reflected with Jaki on this and I learnt that not all women want to engage and not all woman-midwife relationships are the same. I felt very little reward from case-loading this woman, although I did learn a lot from looking after her. Strangely enough, the reward from her came a few months ago when she was being cared for by Jaki during her second pregnancy. When Jaki was on annual leave, the woman asked to see me for her appointment instead of one of the other midwives in the team. It was a small reward, but a reward, nonetheless.

The case load experience was complemented by the academic decision-making module, which really honed my practice and made me consider not only my involvement in women's individual care but also my role in the maternity system. It made me question where my allegiances lie and highlighted the need to be strong-willed, yet professional, when advocating for the women in my care. I learnt that pushing to get women what they want was at the heart of my values, and this is something that I have carried forwards into my practice as a qualified midwife. I love meeting women who make requests that fall outside of guidelines or standard practice and supporting them to achieve the birth preferences and experiences that they want. My practice evolved immensely because of my case load experience, giving me the confidence that I was ready to qualify because I knew that I would never know the answer to all the questions that either myself or the women had, but the case load had enabled me to construct a toolkit of contacts who might be able to help me find those answers.

As a qualified midwife, I love supporting students in practice and the case load experience is one of my favourite times to do this because it means watching women grow and students grow at the same time. Seeing a student realise they can safely, confidently and competently guide a woman from early pregnancy right through to postnatal discharge is a real privilege and I love seeing students' passion as they go through the case load and experience the satisfaction at completing it. Naturally there are challenges and, just as Jaki struggled to relinquish control to me, I struggle to relinquish control to the next generation of students not because I do not trust them, but rather because my antenatal case load is the heart of my own midwifery practice. At present, I do not work in a continuity of carer team due to family circumstances meaning I would be unable to work an on-call roster. That said, I provide continuity of carer to two case loads' of women in the antenatal period, including for women in need of extra support, and we round off their care by discharging our own case loads' of women postnatally. While this is not true continuity, I also work across the midwifery-led and obstetric-led birth environments to provide labour care and so am occasionally able to provide intrapartum care to women in my case load. I can appreciate the impact that continuity has on both women and midwives, and while this impact is largely positive, there are negatives too. Continuity of any kind can be draining because there is always the risk that you begin to carry the weight of the case load, not only in terms of the actual workload, but also in terms of the emotional toll of shouldering the women's stories, problems, mental health concerns, and trauma. The most important thing that having a case load has taught me is the need to have an incredible safety net for the challenging days. I always joke that I have a tribe behind me, but it is true. I have a tribe of incredible friends and colleagues who make me laugh and listen to me rant; I work in a small team who know only too well the challenges and the rewards of community midwifery; my team leader was my mentor as a student and she listens to me talk through my day, she sits back while I pick apart my practice, and watches as I learn and move on (and then I do the same for her); I have a best friend that I like to call my life guru who sees me through the darkest days when I occasionally wonder why I am a midwife.

Midwifery is hard. It is emotionally gruelling, shift work is tiring, women can be draining, but for all the challenges, you are entering into the most incredible profession. The life guru once told me that midwifery is not something you do; it is something you are. When I was a first-year student and found myself struggling, Ellen asked me why I wanted to be a midwife, why all the sacrifices were worth it. She asked me on a particularly bad day and I honestly did not have an answer for her. About eighteen months later, I was struggling to tell my labour ward mentor what my strengths as a student midwife were (I had a dozen or so weaknesses listed for her), so she instead asked me why I wanted to be a midwife. That time, my answer was instant: because I love women. As a qualified midwife, I still hold that thought in my head, I keep it in easy reach because there are always going to be challenges, there will always be days when you feel like you are drowning. Those days are easier if you have a tribe behind you, willing you on, and if you have a reason for doing it. As you begin your case load, and you progress through it, as you meet every single challenge on your road to becoming a midwife, I urge you to remember your motivation. It will make you keep going. For me it was simple, and it still is – because I love women. I want that love and passion for women and midwifery to shine, I want women to feel it, and I want you to own it and to be proud of it.

## Lessons learnt?

As a module lead and academic assessor, the typical challenges presented to me are how students and women say goodbye at the end of the experience. It is pertinent to consider this prior to engaging in any professional relationship. It is a professional relationship, you are not 'friends'; you may be friendly, but you are there for a snapshot in a person's life and experiences. You may require support from your PMA or practice supervisor if this is something you experience.

The sharing of personal phone numbers has proved to be a concern in several situations. There have been scenarios where women complain that they perceive the student to be overzealous or fanatical through continuously phoning them. Equally, women have persistently been calling the student as their personal source of advice and support. There have been cases where the women have left voice mails or text students when experiencing an obstetric emergency rather than phoning the emergency hospital contacts leading to disastrous outcomes due to messages not being dealt with appropriately or in a timely way. Adverse events and investigations have ensued where students have undertaken clinical visits without reporting back their findings to the named midwife and/or undertaking all visits with no qualified practitioner input leading to poor outcomes.

Most feedback concerns the non-attendance at pre-planned appointments with no follow up communication to the midwife or the woman. This has led to some women declining to have the student attend future care episodes with them as they feel let down. Frequently students are not called for the birth and so miss that part of the experience.

## Box 4.4 Vignette 4.2 in Summary

Many years ago, when I was a student midwife, case load experiences were not the norm or expectation. However, as a newly qualified midwife in the late 1990s, the drive was to join a small team of case load held midwives across several areas within the locality. I fully embraced the concept of case load practice and agreed with the findings of greater maternal satisfaction and improved health outcomes for women and their families. At that time in my life, I could not have contemplated this due to be a mother to a young child, having a partner working random long shifts and living 30 miles away from my place of employment. I was not able to commit to working in a truly flexible way to meet the needs of the women covered by the team approach. This did impact negatively upon my conscience and how I perceived my contribution to the team, the women and to the profession.

As I could not commit to the clinical requirements of the case load role, I was able to contribute in an alternative way. I led on the development of a new 'New Deals for Communities' (Department of Environment, Transport and the Regions, 1998) midwifery case-loading project. The plan was to set up and deliver a case load midwifery project with 5.0 whole time equivalent team members covering the 24-hour period, 365 days per year for all antenatal, intra partum and post-partum activities for the case load. The project needed to integrate a multi-agency approach to enhancing the locality through health, education, social and parenting skills. This was an educational and developmental venture for me as I had never written a 'sustainable' long term project with the need to secure funding prior to this. I had been used to writing academic essays using critical appraisal of the evidence base to inform decisions and action as a student. What I had not considered was the fact that the communities reading academically written documents would feel offended by the terminologies used to refer to their 'normality'. I attended community-led development meetings and presented the maternity services project plan alongside my senior manager. I was naive in attending meetings thinking that everyone would be welcoming what we had to offer, but instead we were sent away to re-evaluate our approach to the proposal. Working with the community to develop a project and gain a collective agreement for the funding and future monitoring of outputs has shown me that services cannot 'do to' communities but needs to 'work with' in collaboration to ensure clinical needs and expectations are met.

If I had experienced a case load experience as a student, would it have changed how I approached the project planning experience? This is difficult to answer. The level of my understanding has changed due to the experiences that I have had during my career and at the start of my career I thought I knew much more than I did. My perceptions now from setting up and managing this project and through setting up case load activities for students as part of their pre-registration preparation hopefully shows a level of understanding and practicality but having never worked in this way I am cognisant of my limitations. Students have, over the past ten years of me leading their case load activities, evaluated the experience in a positive way and highlighted areas for their own professional development and consideration of how they can contribute to a case load or, more recently, a continuity of carer model of care. My passion in supporting 'transition' to 'becoming' a midwife (Kitson-Reynolds, 2010) encompasses the realities individuals face and the self-determination required to build resilience to meet the ever-changing clinical workload.

## References

ACT Academy (n.d.). *SBAR Communication Tool: Situation, Background, Assessment, Recommendation.* NHS Improvement. Available at: https://improvement.nhs.uk/documents/2162/sbar-communication-tool.pdf [accessed: 31 December, 2020].

Ashforth, K., & Kitson-Reynolds, E. (2018). Decision-making: Do existing models reflect the complex and multifaceted nature of woman-centred contemporary midwifery practice? Part 1. *The Practising Midwife*, 21(10): 10–13.

Brown, B. (2015). *Rising Strong*. London, Vermillion.

*Data Protection Act 2018*. Available at: www.legislation.gov.uk/ukpga/2018/12/contents/enacted [accessed: 2 December, 2019].

Department of Environment, Transport and the Regions (1998). *New Deal for Communities: Phase 1 Proposals: Guidance for Pathfinder Applicants*. London: DETR.

Gibbs, G. (1988). *Learning by Doing: A Guide to Teaching and Learning Methods*. London: Further Education Unit.

Johns, C. (2009). *Becoming a Reflective Practitioner*, 3rd ed. West Sussex: Wiley-Blackwell.

Kitson-Reynolds, E. (2010). The Lived Experience of Newly Qualified Midwives. Southampton, University of Southampton thesis.

Lewis, A. (2020). Using appreciative inquiry (AI) as a solution focussed approach to organisational change in two educational psychology services. In J. Hardy & M. Bham, (Eds.), *Leadership for Educational Psychologists: Principles and Practicalities*. USA: Wiley Publishers.

Nursing and Midwifery Council (2017). *Revalidation: How to Revalidate with the NMC. Requirements for Renewing your Registration*. London: NMC. Available at: http://revalidation.nmc.org.uk/download-resources/guidance-and-information/ [accessed: 1 September, 2020].

Nursing and Midwifery Council (2018). *Part 2: Standards for Student Supervision and Assessment*. London: NMC.

Nursing and Midwifery Council (2019). *Standards for Pre-Registration Midwifery Programmes*. London: NMC.

Saleebey, D. (Ed.) (2013). *The Strengths Perspective in Social Work Practice*, 6th ed. Boston, MA: Allyn and Bacon.

Schon, D. (1991). *The Reflective Practitioner: How Professionals Think in Action*. Aldershot: Ashgate Publishing Ltd.

# 5 Considerations for practice supervisors, practice assessors and academic assessors

*Marie Naish*

## Introduction

We have explored the considerations students should make in relation to setting up, undertaking and evaluating their case load held practice, but as practice supervisors and assessors you must also explore what student case load held practice means for you, and how you can best support students to achieve their goals. As a practice partner with an Approved Education Institution (AEI), you may also have questions about how best to approach case load held practice, and the responsibilities you have in supporting both students and the practice setting. This chapter provides hints and tips for practice supervisors/assessors, academic assessors and AEIs to support the planning, implementation and evaluation of case load held practices for pre-registration midwifery students. Reading through may present more questions than answers, as there are elements that AEIs and practice partners will need to consider and agree upon together. There is not one agreed way to implement and review case load held practice, however there are principles of best practice to be considered in order to provide clear parameters and guidance for women, students and practice supervisors. Reviewing processes is an important part of midwifery practice, and so while you may already have systems in place, this chapter may provide additional considerations to promote change and adapt the current process.

## A contract

It is best practice to have a contract in place to ensure the parameters of the case load held practice are clear and agreed by all parties, prior to the experience commencing. It is usual for this to be developed and approved by the AEI and practice partner/ Trust in tandem, with service user and student input. Women need to have good understanding of what being part of a student case load means in relation to their maternity care, how they can withdraw from the experience and who they need to contact throughout. For practice supervisors and students, the contract provides an overview of responsibilities and triggers discussion about elements such as the frequency of joint visits.

The contract will include a consent form for the woman, student and practice supervisor to sign before being stored in the woman's notes. It is advised that the consent form includes:

DOI: 10.4324/9781003051527-5

- Contact details for the supervising midwife.
- Generic contact details for the maternity services, should the supervising midwife be unavailable.
- Contact details for the person overseeing the experience at the AEI. This may be the Academic Assessor, or another nominated person.

An example contract, including consent forms, is in Chapter 10.

## Risk assessment

A risk assessment should be undertaken prior to the experience commencing. The risk assessment aims to mitigate against dangers that may present themselves to the student during the case load experience. Like all workplace risk assessments, the document should outline scenarios or hazards that could cause harm, injury or illness to the student and assess the likelihood and seriousness of these hazards, before considering actions that could reduce the likelihood of occurrence (Health and Safety Executive, n.d.). This includes considering the safety of students attending clients houses alone, travelling in the community, both during normal working hours and out of hours, and biohazards associated with the role of a midwife.

It is good practice for the AEI to provide a template risk assessment for students to complete and review with their practice supervisor. An example risk assessment can be found in Chapter 10. Presented below are suggestions for what could be included in the risk assessment however, these may be adapted depending on the nature of the case load experience being undertaken.

### Considering lone working

A lone worker is defined as 'someone who works by themselves without close or direct supervision' (Health and Safety Executive (HSE), 2020). All employers have a responsibility to provide training, supervision and support to lone workers (HSE, 2020). It is possible for students to fall through the gap as they are not usually formally employed by the organisation providing maternity service provision. As part of the experience, students will be working without direct supervision and so it is important that students and supervisors are aware of the local lone working policy to mitigate risk to the student. It is likely students will be venturing out into the community for the first time alone; in previous practice experiences they will have been accompanied by a member of employed staff. Consequently, they may have limited understanding of the local policies regarding lone working. As a practice supervisor you will need to consider:

- What is the lone working policy at the local NHS Trust or organisation?
- How will the policy be applied to student case loading? For example, the lone working policy may state that for out of hours work in the community staff must inform somebody that they have arrived and contact them again to inform them they have left.
- What process does the student need to follow to ensure their safety?
- If there is any further necessary training that the student needs to complete prior to the experience, for example local conflict resolution or lone working training modules.

- Whether the student understands their responsibility to help protect themselves.
- Whether any clients pose additional risk to the student while lone working, and if so, whether lone visits should be undertaken.

### Travelling in the community

Students need to consider their personal safety when travelling alone in the community. Many students will have their own means of transport such as their own car to travel in, however some will rely on walking or public transport to travel to appointments. Discussion regarding how a student intends to get themselves, and the required equipment to appointments and practice, should take place. This is pertinent, as students may not have been 'on call' during the night in previous placements and may not have considered how they can safety travel to the woman's chosen birth location outside of daylight hours. Students should also be reminded to plan their journey, so that they are aware of the route they need to take and any additional considerations such as toll charges.

### Business car insurance

It is likely that most students will use their own vehicle to travel to and from appointments with women and families, and this brings additional considerations for them. Students will need to ensure that they have the relevant car insurance in place, namely business insurance. Providers often offer different levels of business insurance and so it is important that the student checks that they have the appropriate level of cover in place for their activities and to cover the equipment they will carry with them. Of course, it is the responsibility of the student as the driver of a vehicle to ensure that they have the relevant cover, however it can be useful to provide a reminder for them as this may not have been something they have been required to consider before.

### Breakdown cover

Students should ensure that their vehicle is in good working order prior to travelling to case load appointments. This includes ensuring the car is filled with an appropriate amount of fuel for the outgoing and return journey, considering the possibility of any traffic delays. In addition, students are strongly recommended to have breakdown cover in place, to ensure they can be attended to and/or rescued should their vehicle break down and they become stranded in the community. Some AEI/NHS Trusts insist on students having breakdown cover in place for them to attend visits in the community. It would be beneficial to discuss this with the student at the beginning of the case load experience.

If a student were to experience a breakdown or road traffic accident the process they need to follow must be clear. Agree with the student what they must do in this instance, for example report to you as practice supervisor, and the central maternity unit. This not only ensures the safety of the student, but also enables the maternity service to follow up with the family, should the appointment be cancelled or rearranged as a result.

### Methods of communication

In order to adhere to the lone worker policy students will need to carry a charged mobile telephone with them. It is usual for students to use their personal mobile

*Table 5.1* Lone working checklist

| Prior to undertaking any appointments on your own consider the following to help keep yourself safe. | | | | | | | | |
|---|---|---|---|---|---|---|---|---|
| Checklist item | Date | Date | Date | Date | Date | Date | Date | Date |
| Have you informed somebody of the appointment, including location, timing and expected appointment length (as per the lone working policy)? | | | | | | | | |
| Have you provided your vehicle details to somebody who knows where you going? | | | | | | | | |
| Do you have a charged mobile phone on you? | | | | | | | | |
| Have you planned your route to the appointment location? | | | | | | | | |
| Do you have the appropriate car insurance in place? | | | | | | | | |
| Do you have plenty of fuel in your vehicle? | | | | | | | | |
| Do you have breakdown cover in place? | | | | | | | | |

telephone for this. Clarify this with the student, to ensure they have a mobile device and plan they can use to fulfil this. It is advised that it is not assumed that students have a mobile phone, and a plan with unlimited calls, as some may not be in a financial position to afford this. The next step is to provide the student with the emergency numbers they need so that they can enter them into their device. This would include numbers such as your own work telephone number, the community midwives' office and the local maternity centre generic number. Having these numbers saved in the device will mean they are to hand for the student, should they need help, support or advice in a hurry.

Tip: consider making a checklist for students to refer to prior to each lone working appointment, as seen in Table 5.1.

### Biohazards

As a qualified member of staff, and employee at an organisation, you will be familiar with the processes and policies in place to deal with any biohazards and the management of clinical waste. While students will have training and experience in these areas, it is unlikely that prior to case load experience that they will have carried biohazards and clinical waste themselves in the community. Providing the organisational policies to the student, and explaining the process you undertake yourself, will support the student in undertaking this new responsibility. Students will need to be provided with the organisation's clinical waste bags, and a portable sharps container, and informed to always carry these with them when working in a community setting.

*Equipment*

All equipment used by students must be approved and tested by the organisation. It is the organisation's responsibility to ensure that equipment is provided to care for women accessing maternity care, and that the equipment is safe to use. The organisation is provided with the funding to deliver care to women, including the provision of equipment, and as such equipment need not be provided by the AEI. As practice supervisor you will need to support the student in obtaining suitable equipment to enable them to provide the necessary care. You may find that some AEIs provide bags for the students to use, often on a rotational basis, however the equipment held within them must come from the organisation providing the care.

Prior to the experience it is beneficial to discuss with the student what equipment they will need, how they will ensure it is suitable and how much stock to carry, to ensure they are not wasting equipment. Students undertaking case load experience should be aware of the importance of ensuring equipment is in date and, if required, tested regularly, but reminding them of these aspects will support their learning and transition to an autonomous practitioner. Students are reminded that the equipment for appointments is funded through the NHS and therefore only the equipment needed for the visit must be taken. Students are reminded of the need to be resource savvy.

## Deciding whether to supervise a student's case load practice

**Box 5.1  Activity 5.1**

Let us set the scene – a student midwife you worked with during their first year of training approaches you and asks you to supervise their case load practice. What considerations should you make before deciding to support the student?

- Has the student provided you with enough information about what supervising this experience would entail?
- Have you discussed with the student their expectations of you, and yours of them?
- How will you communicate in a tripartite way, involving yourself, the woman and student?
- Have you assessed the student to be competent to undertake lone visits?
- Do you have good communication channels set up with the student?
- Have you agreed a process to follow should they unexpectedly be unable to attend an appointment?
- Are you confident that the student will report back to you accurately following the visit?

## Professional responsibility

As the midwife responsible for the woman's care the student you are supporting will be working under your professional registration. This may seem daunting but remember you should not agree to supervise a student's case load practice if you do not assess them to be competent to provide care under indirect supervision, including the undertaking of lone visits. The AEI and NHS organisation will negotiate together to agree a suitable point in the midwifery curriculum that student case load held practice is appropriate, however readiness will differ for individual students. It should be considered what exposure to clinical practice the student has had to date, and in which clinical areas. As the registrant you remain responsible and accountable for the woman's care, as per the NMC (2015) Code, and as such you are advised to observe the care provided by student midwives prior to agreeing to supervise their experience.

A few questions you may like to ask yourself regarding your professional responsibly include:

- What is your responsibility to the woman and family as a registrant?
- How often are you going to see the woman yourself?
- How are you going to supervise the student when you are not physically present?
- What information do you want the student to provide following a lone visit?
- How will you record the discussions that you have with the student and any decisions made?
- How will you ensure the woman and/or family can raise any concerns about their care with you?
- What contingency plan is in place if the student unexpectantly cannot attend an appointment?

### Box 5.2 Activity 5.2

*Case study*

A student midwife provided care for a woman and her family during the antenatal period as part of their case load experience. The woman intended to birth her baby at the stand-alone birth centre. On admission in labour at 40 weeks gestation, the midwife working alongside the student identified that the symphysis-fundal height was outside the expected parameters. On review of the notes, it was clear that static growth had not been detected during antenatal visits conducted by the student midwife, and as a result the relevant guideline had not been followed. The woman had last seen a qualified midwife at 28 weeks' gestation. The student had verbally reported to the midwife supervising the experience that fetal growth was normal. The woman was transferred to the hospital for labour and diagnosed with intrauterine growth restriction.

*Analysis of case study*

Case studies such as this can be anxiety inducing and deter midwives from wanting to supervise students undertaking lone visits. Rather than discourage you, it is presented to demonstrate why considering your professional responsibilities and boundaries are so important. Undertaking alternate visits with the student would have enabled the midwife to review previous symphysis-fundal height measurements and identify static growth. The supervisor could also have asked the student to be more specific with their verbal update after each lone visit, providing the symphysis-fundal height measurement for the midwife to log. You may think of other ideas to support midwives in monitoring the care provided, but as a minimum it is recommended that the midwife responsible attends alternate antenatal and postnatal community visits, and all labour assessments.

## Inviting women to participate in student case load held practice

Once you have agreed to supervise a student undertaking case load practice the next step is to identify women to invite to participate. There are no exclusions to the women that students can case load – only those that decline to participate. Students can case load vulnerable women and women with complex medical needs, but your involvement and attendance in these cases may be increased. For example, if a student arranges to case load a woman with significant safeguarding concerns, whereby lone visits are not appropriate, you would need to attend each appointment with the student as per the policy.

The best starting place when deciding who to invite is to ask the student what they want to achieve through their case load experience. They may identify a group of women with whom they have had limited exposure to or experience with to date. It is beneficial for students to case load women with a mix of requirements, for example women with uncomplicated pregnancies, women aiming for vaginal birth after cae-sarean section or with multiple pregnancy, and women with complex social or medical needs. This mix enables the student to experience the differences in providing con-tinuity of carer to women from a range of backgrounds and with differing needs. This can be a beneficial learning experience for students as they come to know the processes required for a range of scenarios. Often students, though competent in their clinical care by the point of taking a case load of women, have limited understanding and experiences of the 'behind the scenes' processes, referrals and communications the midwife undertakes with a range of professionals and services. Providing a case load that exposes the students to a range of processes is therefore enriching to their development.

Once it has been explored with the student what they want to achieve through the experience, the next step is to invite the women to participate in the student case load held experience. The responsible midwife should discuss the option of student case load held practice with the woman, explaining that it is entirely her choice whether to agree to the experience. The midwife will outline the parameters of the experience, how the student would be monitored in the care provided and what changes to her care may result from participating. It can be beneficial for women and students to meet at an appointment with the named midwife, prior to the woman being invited to participate. This allows opportunity for women to form their own assessment of the student and helps them consider their choice to participate in case load held practice.

## Communication

Clear communication channels are required for the case load experience to be successful. All involved parties need to be aware of the channels agreed, and circumstances in which to use them. Considerations need to be made regarding communication between women and students, women and practice supervisors, students and practice supervisors and with the AEI. Women must be clear about who they need to contact if they require help or advice during the experience. The process for this is likely to differ, depending on your agreed practice; some AEIs advise against the student providing a direct means of communication for women to contact them, for example by giving the woman their personal mobile phone number. The student will be attending practice learning environments and theory teaching, and therefore may be unavailable to respond to contact from the woman. Providing a personal mobile phone number would not allow for the same voicemail message to women and their families needing help, as required for employed midwives. This could lead to women not being informed of what to do in an emergency and not seeking further support, but instead waiting for the student to contact them. All parties must remain aware that the student is not yet a registered practitioner, and as such needs to be supervised in their practice. This does not prevent the student from speaking with, or seeing women, without the practice supervisor present, but careful consideration would need to be made regarding in what circumstances it would be appropriate for women to contact the student directly.

Different challenges present when the woman does not have a contact number for the student. These include:

- The student not being updated regarding a change of appointment time/location.
- The student not being informed when the woman is admitted for labour assessment.
- The student not being updated to changes to the care plan following unscheduled episodes of care they have not attended.

To help prevent these challenges occurring, consider ways for the student to be updated. Some organisations implement a sticker for the front of the woman's hand-held notes indicating they have consented to student case load held practice, which student is supporting them and when to contact the student. Of course, the environment the woman attends would need access to the student's personal mobile phone number, and as such these should be stored somewhere convenient, yet secure, for clinicians to access when they need to contact the student.

It should also be considered what opportunities women have, to communicate with the midwife without the student present. Women need to be aware how to raise any concerns they may have about their care, and an open dialogue with the supervising midwife. Women must be aware that they can withdraw from the experience at any point but agreeing a regular timeline of communication with women and their families can prevent issues arising and help resolve them swiftly if they do. Communication between women and practice supervisors also allows opportunity to gather feedback on the students practice and progress from the family's perspective.

## Communication between the student, midwife and AEI

While communication between the woman and care providers is key, it is also important to discuss how the student, midwife and AEI will communicate. The following questions should be considered:

- How does the midwife know the student has an appointment with the woman?
- What happens if the midwife is on annual leave? Who does the student report to instead?
- How do the midwife and student communicate after the appointment? How quickly does this happen? It is advised that any care episodes or interactions with women that are not directly supervised by the midwife are reported as soon as possible. This allows the care plan to be discussed and amended if necessary, in a timely manner.
- How does the student ensure they can contact the midwife during the appointment?
- What communication lines are set up between the student, midwife and AEI?
- How does the student record their experience?

## Attendance

Outlining the parameters of the case load held experience right at the start of the process is important to ensure agreement between AEIs, practice partners and students regarding the expectations of students. One area of consideration is attendance. Students are required to balance the case load experience with their usual programme requirements, with it likely that they will be undertaking the experience while also attending clinical placements and/or taught University content. A study by McLachlan et al. (2013), conducted in Australia, found that 97% of midwifery academics reported that case load held practice impacted student attendance at University sessions. As an AEI and organisation providing maternity care, you may want to agree some principles to present to the students when introducing the experience; to reduce the likelihood that either practice learning, or theory learning becomes heavily prioritised. Considerations may be as follows:

- How much care do you anticipate students should provide? Students should not be able to select parts of care they want to be involved in, and opt out of care episodes they are less interested in. Part of the experience is understanding the commitment required for case load held practice however there may be practical elements to consider, such as student annual leave entitlement, attendance at mandatory teaching sessions and family commitments.
- Do students attend antenatal or postnatal appointments for women over attending AEI taught content? Or are students expected to work appointments around AEI taught content?
- Are students on call for the woman's labour and birth?
- What happens if the woman starts labour before or during AEI taught content? Does the student attend?
- How will students demonstrate that they have completed the taught content if they miss a session to attend a case load clinical experience?

- If a student is on placement in one clinical area, are they able to leave that area to attend a case load experience elsewhere? If so, what process would they need to follow to enable them to do this?
- How will you ensure students are working within the EU Working Time Directive?

## Clinical hours

While not technically employed by the NHS or AEI, students are usually expected to work within the Governments maximum weekly working hours, meaning they cannot work more than 48 hours per week as averaged over 17 weeks (Gov.UK, n.d.). As an AEI you might like to consider whether the delivery of taught content, and self-directed study, would count towards these working hours when delivered alongside the case load held practice experience.

Pre-registration midwifery education programmes with NMC approval will have an equal split of 50% theory and 50% practice learning (NMC, 2019). To avoid students working unnecessarily long hours, as an AEI you could consider integrating the case load held experience into a programme module, allocating practice learning time and credit to the experience.

It is imperative that students are not attending clinical placements when they are not fit to attend, including due to tiredness or fatigue. Students must be aware of their limitations and the necessity to look after their health in order to protect the public. An example would be that a student who has worked a night shift, supporting a woman and family during labour, should not then attend a full day at University, or vice versa, with no adequate time between to rest and recuperate. While this can be frustrating for students, potentially leading them to miss valuable case load held experiences, it is a learning process for them to understand the dilemmas and responsibilities presented with on call midwifery practice.

## Documentation

Record keeping is integral to the midwife's role and a requirement of the NMC (2015) Code to maintain contemporaneous records. Prior to the student commencing case load practice it is recommended a discussion around documentation takes place. For the student to undertake lone visits you must be confident that they can document their visit, assessment and decisions appropriately and in line with NMC guidance. It is good practice to ensure you are visiting the woman at every other appointment with the student, providing regular opportunity to review and discuss documentation. This should give the opportunity to countersign previous entries.

A more complex issue is that of electronic records. There are differing practices between organisations with regards to whether students are given credentials to access electronic records. It would be wise to review this as an organisation and decide the best way forward with regards to the support provided to students. It is likely, if students themselves do not have access, that the responsible midwife will need to input any electronic records. It is imperative that a student accessing records after an employee has logged in using their credentials is directly overseen in this activity. Part of the learning activity for students is to gain understanding of the administration related to the role of the midwife, and so it is important that they are exposed and encouraged to learn about processes and systems under supervision.

## The organisation and follow up of clinical investigations

NHS Trust policy usually stipulates that the professional taking and requesting an investigation has responsibility for following up the result. Practice supervisors and students need to review the policy at their organisation and consider whether agreement is in place for students to place requests. Often, particularly if such requests are made digitally, an employed registrant is the only person able to submit requests and access results. Whether the student can complete this task or not, as the supervising midwife responsible for the woman's care, you must follow up on investigations, and the actions resulting from those investigations.

The challenge comes in supporting the student to develop skills in this area if they do not have access to the relevant systems to request and follow up investigations. Case load held practice enables the student to experience the 'behind the scenes' activities that often a practice supervisor will undertake while the student is elsewhere. Without exposure to these tasks, on qualification students can be shocked at the amount of administration and follow up required for the midwife's role. If students are unable to personally submit the request or follow up the results, they can still be involved in the process. Between you, agree a way that this activity can happen while you are working together. While the student may not be able to access blood or scan results, they can be provided with the results for them to interpret, relay the findings to the woman and form any necessary management plan.

## Measuring success

Case load held practice is a new, exciting and yet daunting prospect for midwifery students. It is imperative that they receive regular feedback on their progress and success. There are multiple ways this can be achieved such as:

- Collating feedback from women and families regarding their experience including what went well, what could be improved, any areas to commend the student on and/or areas of concern.
- Undertaking tripartite reviews with:

  a  The woman, student and practice supervisor
  b  The student, practice supervisor and AEI
  c  The student, practice supervisor and practice assessor

- Regular updating between student and midwife.
- Completion of a daily log by the student; documenting activity and learning.
- Alternate visits with the midwife for the student's practice to be observed.
- Completion of regular reflections on practice by student.
- Completion of an associated assessment activity, if part of their curriculum.

## Case loading friends and family

Rarely, a student may request to case load a friend or family member – so what happens here?

It is best to check the organisation policy, to ensure good understanding of the process for an employee wanting to care for a relation or friend. This will provide you with knowledge about the approvals and paperwork, if any, required in this circumstance. Furthermore, this is a good learning opportunity for the student to gain better understanding of the process and considerations needed in these cases ready for qualification. It is also advised that discussion takes place with the AEI, as it may be that they have, or want to have, a policy that does not permit students to care for friends and family.

It would be wise to explore with the student their motivation for wanting to provide case load held care to a friend or family member and discuss the pros and cons to this experience. It might be beneficial to link with a tutor at the AEI, or Professional Midwifery Advocate, to explore this in depth. The student should be encouraged to consider:

- What are the expectations of the friend or family member of them?
- How would the student ensure they are still supervised by a qualified practitioner if offering support and guidance informally to the pregnant person or family?
- What happens if the pregnancy or birth outcome is poor, or if the care does not go according to plan?
- How would the student feel if the case load experience negatively affected the relationship with the friend or family member?
- How would the student ensure that they can meet their other responsibilities and training requirements alongside case loading a friend or family member?
- What other options might be possible? For example, the student taking the role of a birth partner, or attending appointments as a friend in a non-professional manner.

If the organisation and AEI both confirm it is appropriate for a student to offer a case load held experience to a friend or family, and the student has had the opportunity to explore the questions above, the next step would be to explore the option with the woman and family. It is necessary to provide the same information about being part of a student case load as you would to any woman, however there may be additional considerations in this case such as:

- Ensuring the parameters of the student case load, and the role of the supervising midwife, are explicitly clear to ensure the student is not put in a compromising position.
- Exploring how the woman and family may feel if the outcome of the pregnancy or birth is poor, or the care does not go according to plan.
- Discussing the potential implications of outcomes on the long-term relationship between the family and student.

## In summary

This chapter has provided practice supervisors, assessors and AEIs with areas for consideration when implementing student case load held practice. We have explored the practicalities of preparing students for lone working, how to decide whether to supervise a student undertaking an experience and how best to ensure good communication channels between families, students and supervisors. Key considerations as a registrant have been discussed, including in relation to professional responsibility, and the practicalities of delivering care in this model explored.

# References

Gov.UK (n.d.). Maximum weekly working hours. Available at: www.gov.uk/maximum-week ly-working-hours [accessed: 30 November, 2020].

Health and Safety Executive (2020). Protecting lone workers. How to manage the risks of working alone. Available at: www.hse.gov.uk/pubns/indg73.pdf [accessed: 30 November, 2020].

Health and Safety Executive (n.d.). Managing risks and risk assessment at work. Available at: www.hse.gov.uk/simple-health-safety/risk/index.htm [accessed: 30 November, 2020].

McLachlan, H.L., Newton, M., Nightingale, H., Morrow, J., & Kruger, G. (2013). Exploring the 'follow-through experience': A statewide survey of midwifery students and academics conducted in Victoria, Australia. *Midwifery*, 29(9): 1064–1072.

Nursing and Midwifery Council (2015). *The Code: Standards of Conduct, Performance and Ethics for Nurses and Midwives.* London: NMC.

Nursing and Midwifery Council (2019). *Standards for Pre-Registration Midwifery Programmes.* London: NMC.

# 6 The emotional aspects of continuity of carer

*Kate Ashforth and Emer Kelly*

## Introduction

The case load held or continuity of carer experience is intended as a learning journey situated within the real world of midwifery practice that prepares you with the requisite skills for transition to qualified status (Fry et al., 2013). Exposing you to the case load held experience goes beyond technical skill acquisition and aims to instil an appreciation of the art of midwifery, and an ability to develop a trusting woman-midwife relationship that incorporates advocacy and collaboration (Browne et al., 2014). Furthermore, it enables students generally to step beyond their current role and into the shoes of a qualified midwife, having an increased sense of responsibility and autonomy while still practising within their scope of practice, supported by midwives (Fry et al., 2013; Rawnson, 2011). The experience facilitates you to care for a small case load of women holistically across the childbirth continuum and, while the literature has examined the student experience of continuity of carer, both as a case load and as part of practice placements within small continuity of carer teams, it has failed to examine the emotional journey that students undergo while caring for their case load. As such, this chapter considers the emotional journey of the continuity of carer experience and examines the literature base of confidence and competence; professional boundaries and responsibilities; work-life balance; human factors; resilience and burnout; future practice. The chapter includes vignettes of student and midwife voices to lend authenticity to an otherwise under-explored area of practice in current literature.

> **Box 6.1 Vignette 6.1**
>
> Having no previous clinical experience, and an inner critic that loved to wax lyrical about my perceived shortcomings, I spent a lot of my training feeling inadequate and out of my depth, which was compounded by the fact that my peers seemed to love every minute of midwifery. Then came my 'wow moment'. My community mentor, Jaki, and I crept into a woman's birth room in the darkest hour of the night to give her midwife a break. Fairy lights were dotted around the room and the woman was tranquil in the pool. At one point she looked up, fear and uncertainty haunted her eyes as her body began to move and swell with the intensity of labour. Jaki was with her in an instant, crouching down, cupping the woman's face in her hands and locking eyes with her. I've been subject to that look myself a few times over the years, it instils confidence when it is most needed and it tells you that you are enough, just as you

DOI: 10.4324/9781003051527-6

are. That look was one of love, kindness, tenderness and compassion, but it was also one of absolute confidence, strength, protection and loyalty. The moment shared by Jaki and the woman blew me away, it was the moment that I saw the midwife I wanted to become and subsequently I spent a lot of my training honing my skills to become my version of that midwife. Placements ebbed and flowed: community shifts blended into labour ward, a birth centre rotation flowed into the postnatal ward, and the middle of my second year saw the beginning of my continuity of carer experience. Continuity of carer felt as though I was building a toolkit for future practice and it gave me the opportunity to connect with myself as a midwife, and it made me examine my values and my practice even more closely than previously. I was confident discussing my clinical reasoning and decision-making with Jaki, as the midwife supervising my case load, and we had always reflected extensively on practice. Furthermore, she pushed me to become the midwife she always knew I would be, challenging my presuppositions and thinking in a constructive manner. She had high expectations of me because she wanted me to reach my potential, to provide the best possible care to each woman, to learn from and connect with the experience, and to feel proud of how much I had achieved. Continuity of carer was hard work but rewarding, and it was a culmination of everything I had learned so far. It was never about box-ticking, it was about building a relationship with a case load of women and feeling like a real midwife. One of the biggest challenges was the realisation that sometimes those relationships are not reciprocal, and you do not get the validation you feel you deserve, yet even though the relationships you build with each woman can be different, the care you give to each woman is equal. Signing a continuity of carer contract with Jaki and each woman was the way we gained the woman's consent to participate, but it was also a statement of my commitment to my mentor and to the woman. It was a promise to take part in her care to the best of my ability, to the full extent that she deserved, to involve Jaki in the care, to feedback to her. It was a pledge to travel the woman's journey alongside her or right behind her, and it was Jaki's pledge to support me through that journey. It was an acknowledgment of the importance and the privilege to be allowed to share it with the woman, and it is that commitment that I want students undertaking their continuity of carer with me to understand.

## Confidence and competence

Midwifery education prepares you to be safe, competent and effective practitioners (NMC, 2010) and curricula are responsive to changes in service provision and demographics. Continuity of carer, as delineated in Domain Two of the new standards for midwifery education (NMC, 2019), is one such development. You will be given the opportunity to work in ways that advocate continuity of carer throughout your training, one such way may be case loading a small number of women, either on an individual or group basis. The case load held experience aims to increase confidence and competence in providing continuity of carer and holistic, woman-centred care across the childbirth continuum (Corrigan, 2017), transcending the boundaries of community and hospital-based care. you are expected to follow the woman for whom you are providing care across the spectrum of care environments, determined by the woman's wishes and the clinical picture. As such, care may occur in community-based clinics, birth centres, delivery suite, obstetric clinics, or at home, and you are presumed to be able to move seamlessly and willingly from one to another. Community and hospital-based midwifery are thought to embody two distinct pervading ideologies of mid-wifery practice. While community midwifery advocates an individualised 'with woman' model of care, hospital-based practice leans towards a medicalised 'with institution' model, and this conflict of ideologies is thought to be the main source of emotion work in midwifery (Hunter, 2004). The level of emotional dissonance experienced may be increased due to the reality of practice being inconsistent with personal beliefs about care (Blomberg & Sahlberg-Blom, 2007), which may have a negative effect on your own well-being (Zapf, 2002). The case load held experience reiterates the importance of prioritising people by developing meaningful relationships with the case load women (NMC, 2015; Corrigan, 2017), and the role of the student in an institution-focused model of care with fragmented provision of carer may be to advocate even more vociferously and ensure the woman's voice does not get lost in procedure-driven care. The conflicting ideologies of midwifery practice may be particularly problematic for novice practitioners, such as students, to navigate (Hunter, 2004).

Students generally may be supervised by one midwife during the antenatal period because care is provided for women originally allocated to that midwife's case load, yet the ad hoc allocation of midwives to care for women during labour may increase student stress (Sidebotham & Fenwick, 2019; Ashforth, 2020). Working alongside, or being supervised by, midwives who are unknown to both you and the woman may inhibit your confidence to care and advocate for women: a trusting relationship between the woman and you, and between the you and the midwife, is instrumental to your learning (Sidebotham & Fenwick, 2019). Continuity of supervising midwife across the case load held practice continuum may allow for increased learning opportunities and enable you to analyse and reflect upon your practice and identify as a future midwife (Sweet & Glover, 2013). This could be facilitated by you undertaking your case load experience within a continuity of carer team, meaning you would provide labour care alongside a member of the team within which you are working. The number of women receiving care in continuity of carer teams is not yet sufficient to enable all students to case load in this way. Those students who did work in a continuity of carer model of care reported increased levels of confidence, independence and skill acquisition, in turn bridging the theory-practice gap, when compared with placements in non-case load models (Gray et al., 2013; Browne et al., 2014; Fenwick et al., 2018; Sidebotham & Fenwick, 2019). That said, it has been reported that midwives supervising students during their case load act as gatekeepers and intrude upon the student's relationship with the woman for whom they are caring (McKellar et al., 2014; Ashforth, 2020). These findings echo earlier literature that described the controlling hands or guiding hands of midwives with whom students work (Hughes & Fraser, 2011). While guiding hands nurture, coach and encourage students, providing a source of support when needed, but enabling students to fully engage in care and to develop their own professional identity, controlling hands inhibit student practice and dominate the woman-student-midwife relationship (Hughes & Fraser, 2011). Clinical learning during the continuity of carer experience is based on and in authentic situations, although there may be limited opportunities for mentoring or coaching from midwife to student, particularly as the experience progresses and you gain autonomy, and the quality of your experience may depend on the supervising midwife, which can be positive or negative (Ashforth, 2020). When developed to form a trusting relationship, the rapport you have with your supervising midwife should facilitate a valuable learning environment, optimise learning experiences, and increase your confidence (Moncrieff et al., 2020).

---

**Box 6.2 Activity 6.1**

- How do you intend to achieve a balance in the student-woman-midwife relationship, and how do you think you would feel if you felt unable to participate fully in the relationship?
- Reflect on the relationships you have had with practice supervisors, what has been positive and negative about these? What is important to you about the way you work with midwives in practice, what helps you learn and progress?
- How can you bring these positive aspects to the case load to make the experience as beneficial to you as a learning experience as possible?

---

## Professional boundaries and responsibilities

While the case load held practice experience is intended to highlight the realities of working as an autonomous practitioner, there are variations in the level of autonomy that students are given during this experience (Fry et al., 2013). The standards for education to which universities must adhere do not describe the level of supervision required, the number of consecutive appointments that a woman can be seen by a student unsupervised by a midwife, or how discussions between the student and supervising midwife outside of the appointment about the woman's care are to be documented, and this guidance is determined by the individual universities and Trusts (Fry et al., 2013; NMC, 2019). The level of direct supervision by a midwife is also determined by the confidence, competence, and proximity to qualification of the student, and thus direct supervision should be gradually replaced by indirect supervision as the student progresses through the continuity of carer experience and through their training (Rawnson et al., 2009; Fry et al., 2013) (see also Chapter 5). This calls into question the timing of the continuity of carer experience: students may intend to recruit their case load of women towards the end of their second year of training, with this journey spanning the rest of that year and across their third and final year. One study described a model of continuity of carer experiences that spanned the entire training programme (Jefford et al., 2020). Students followed the care of a small case load of women across each year of study, allowing even junior students to experience and appreciate the childbirth journey from beginning to end. Initially, the role of the student was largely observational and developed over the course to become participatory with direct supervision and then enabling them to become the lead care provider with minimal, indirect supervision. While first-year students' role in the woman's care was limited, their commitment to the case load was high and they sought to attend every appointment. Conversely, third-year students were able to participate more fully in the care, but they struggled to juggle such competing demands associated with the completion of the programme as dissertations, final placements, and examinations. The timing of the continuity of carer experience may be pertinent as it may be intended to coincide with academic modules relating to decision-making, autonomous practice, and future professional practice (Ashforth & Kitson-Reynolds, 2019a; Ashforth & Kitson-Reynolds, 2019b). Such modules may prepare students for the continuity of carer experience by encouraging consideration of accountability, scope of practice, role and responsibilities, and this may be formalised into a handbook that provides students with a reference guide to be used during the experience (Rawnson et al., 2009; McKellar et al., 2014). This handbook may provide guidance about professional boundaries, including caring for friends and family whereby mechanisms to protect students caring for women known to them need to exist in line with those for qualified midwives. One Australian study found that students often recruited friends and family to their case load due to the difficulties encountered in recruitment (McKellar et al., 2014), which blurs the line between personal commitments and professional roles and boundaries. The appropriateness of students recruiting women to their own case load must be questioned, and it must be considered whether the supervising midwife is a more appropriate person to do this.

Clear professional boundaries are intended to safeguard the student, the woman, and the supervising midwife. Anecdotally, some midwives do not want the responsibility of supervising a student continuity of carer experience as they feel the student would be practising under their pin, but without direct supervision. The NMC (2019) standards for pre-registration midwifery programmes advocate that students develop the confidence and competence to practice as if qualified during their final year of study. This was transition to their new roles as registrants should be less of a reality shock (Kramer, 1974). When discussing this concept with colleagues, some expressed concern that they would be held accountable for any possible mistakes made by students visiting women without direct supervision. While clear and open lines of communication between the students and supervising midwife are critical in identifying any concerns and ensuring appropriate referrals are made in a timely manner, this may not be watertight. For example, if the symphysis-fundal height is measured incorrectly, a growth-restricted baby may not be detected, which may jeopardise outcomes. A student may report their measurement to the midwife, and no referral made based on this. Colleagues have reported feeling scared that even one unsupervised appointment could be detrimental to the woman and/or baby, and to the midwife herself, with some feeling as though their professional registration would be under threat if such a mistake were made. This once again calls into question timing of student case load held practice experience, competence of the student, and the confidence of the student and that of the midwife in the student. It also highlights the potential need for the supervising midwife to have already worked with the student so that they already know the student's competence and skill level, and that there is a level of trust in the student-midwife relationship, thus enabling the midwife and student to decide the level of supervision that is appropriate.

Professional boundaries and responsibilities need to be established, not just between the student and the supervising midwife, but also between the student, midwife and woman. Students are often seen to go above and beyond standard midwifery care during their continuity of carer experience, calling into question whether the care reflects usual midwifery care and whether this nurtures women's often high expectations of students as care providers (McKellar et al., 2014; Stulz et al., 2020). Some students have reportedly tried to befriend the women in their case load in order to ensure they are invited to attend the birth (McKellar et al., 2014), which could cause questions to arise as to the students' motives for developing close relationships with the woman. While continuity of carer is a practical component of training aimed at giving students the opportunity to experience the full role and scope of midwifery practice (NMC, 2019), it must be conducted appropriately and safely, and must benefit the woman or at least not expose her to substandard care. The outcomes of the student continuity of carer experience for the women should mirror those for women cared for in a continuity of carer model of care by qualified midwives and students should consider their role in facilitating these improved outcomes for women. Clear professional boundaries also protect against burnout as they mean midwives understand their professional role and have mechanisms to create boundaries between their professional and personal lives (Cummins et al., 2017), which students should aim to replicate. In New Zealand, where case loading is well-established, midwives discuss the model of care with the woman from the outset to enable understanding of what the midwife can and cannot offer, and the limit is of their availability, which establishes professional boundaries and realistic expectations (Fereday & Oster, 2010; Gilkison et al., 2015; Moncrieff et al., 2020).

---

**Box 6.3 Activity 6.2**

- What professional boundaries do you think it is important to have in place to protect you, the woman and the supervising midwife during the case load? Think about points mentioned above, and add any others that you think are relevant.
- Think about your responsibilities as a student towards the case load and think about the midwife's responsibilities towards you and the woman. What will you take responsibility for, for example checking blood results, and what will the midwife take responsibility for? What is realistic for you to be able to achieve?

---

## Work-life balance

The sustainability of working in a continuity of carer model of midwifery care depends on midwives being able to manage expectations between themselves and women, for example women knowing how to escalate concerns when their named midwife is not at work or is unavailable (Styles et al., 2020), and students need to manage expectations similarly to protect against burnout during their continuity of carer experience. Students may not always carry mobile phones specifically for their case load to contact them on between appointments, which aims to safeguard women and the student by ensuring concerns are escalated appropriately and not via the student. While this is intended as a safety mechanism, it may also protect against burnout as it limits the contact between the woman and the student to the appointments. Conversely, this may be a factor that limits the authenticity of the continuity of carer experience as the woman may instead contact the supervising midwife, who may inadvertently become the woman's point of reference, which may in turn ostracise the student from the relationship and cause them to disengage from the case load. As such, careful consideration needs to be taken by the woman, student and midwife to ensure that communication is safe, authentic and does not alienate the student.

The continuity of carer experience has been described as stressful and difficult to manage (Gray et al., 2013; McLachlan et al., 2013), not least because of the commitment to be on-call for women during labour and birth, which can reasonably be expected to span from 37 to 42 weeks' gestation. It could be questioned whether this is achievable or sustainable, even for a limited period of time with a limited number of women. The philosophy of continuity of carer, and student provision of this, poses a conflict with other personal, professional and academic commitments, and students must learn to negotiate safe working times with adequate rest in between in order to practise safely and to avoid burnout (Fry et al., 2013). Shift leaders and the midwives with whom students are working need to take responsibility for making sure students do not work beyond usual working hours, and students themselves must be accountable for their own working hours and ability to work safely, even if this means missing out on facilitating a birth or disappointing a woman by having to go home to rest. On-calls, which are integral to continuity of carer (Rawnson et al., 2009), are considered to blur professional boundaries and risk causing burnout, characterised by disturbed sleep, feelings of stress, and diminished passion for midwifery (Homer et al., 2008).

Midwives may struggle with weekly on-call shifts and a case load of women with potentially complex care needs (Collins et al., 2010; Browne et al., 2014), and continuity of carer models of care may offer protective factors to mitigate against these triggers for burnout (Dawson et al., 2018). Increased autonomy, a level of flexibility that allows midwives to arrange their workload around their lives, close relationships forged between women and midwives, and working in a small team of midwives with a shared philosophy of care means midwives working in continuity of carer models reports lower levels of personal and work-related burnout, and higher levels of job satisfaction than those working in non- continuity of carer models (Dawson et al., 2018; Sidebotham & Fenwick, 2019; Styles et al., 2020; Wentworth, 2020). Women also reported that when they receive continuity of carer, their midwife went above and beyond, gave them more time and attention, and made them feel more confident, loved and supported (Allen et al., 2017), although it has been suggested that continuity of carer raises women's expectations and midwives worry about disappointing them (Wentworth, 2020).

Students who undertake a clinical placement in a continuity of carer team may feel more able to see and appreciate the role of the midwife in its entirety, including all the work behind the scenes such as administration and referrals (Sidebotham & Fenwick, 2019; Styles et al., 2020). Similarly, the student continuity of carer experience is an opportunity to not only learn about the full scope of midwifery practice across the childbirth continuum, but also to learn how to manage factors that may contribute to burnout. Thorough planning and preparation may enable students to manage challenges to the case load (Rawnson et al., 2009), for example setting aside specific study time to ensure academic deadlines and obligations continue to be met, or organising childcare. Some students, however, may choose to manage the competing demands of their case load held practice, academic workload, and other life commitments, by interacting intermittently with the women in their case load, although this undermines the authenticity of the experience and the student's commitment to it (Sweet & Glover, 2013). You may feel that the case load held experience has limited significance to you career if you do not aspire to work in a continuity of carer model (Sweet & Glover, 2013). That said, this experience is considered to be positive and promotes personal growth and transformation (Siebold, 2015; Aune et al., 2011). Furthermore, roles that enable the establishment of meaningful woman-midwife relationships are key in building a sustainable midwifery workforce (Sullivan et al., 2011; Pugh et al., 2013).

**Box 6.4 Activity 6.3**

- Have you ever experienced stress of burnout, either during your midwifery training or in another aspect of your life? What caused this, how did you feel, and how did you manage it?
- What other commitments in your life might impact on your case load?
- How can you achieve work-life balance?

**Box 6.5 Vignette 6.2: Emma, a third-year student midwife who has finished her case load experience**

Case loading as a student was a wonderful opportunity. Experiencing first-hand how midwife-client relationships can be strengthened through case-loading put publications like Better Births into context and reinforced for me the importance of developing a case-loading based system of care. Case loading also offered me a first taste of the responsibilities that go with autonomous practice, but in a safe and supervised way. However, being on call from 37–42 weeks for each of my clients impacted my work-life balance dramatically, whether missing my day off to attend a client in labour or rescheduling my anniversary for a client's induction. Case loading taught me resilience, as I learned to adapt my life to an on-call schedule but could make work (particularly alongside study) feel unrelenting at times.

## Commitment and expectations

Traditional practice placements provide a fragmented view of midwifery care (Lewis et al., 2013) and the pervading model of standard care, as opposed to continuity of carer, may not adequately prepare students for their continuity of carer experience. Students do not always have the opportunity to work in a continuity of carer team whereby on-call shifts are the norm, therefore their expectations may be misaligned with the realities of continuity of carer. While the experience is intended to enable students to build meaningful relationships with the women in their care and to gain an understanding of the responsibilities involved in providing care across the childbirth continuum, the level of involvement is not mandated by the UK education standards (NMC, 2019). Primiparous women may be seen by a midwife up to ten times for standard antenatal care in the UK, while multiparas at low risk of complications may be seen up to eight times, and women may receive a minimum of two or three postnatal visits depending on the clinical situation (National Institute for Health and Care Excellence (NICE), 2019).

The current UK standards for midwifery education do not specify how many women in their case load a student must undertake, nor do they delineate what constitutes continuity of carer in terms of the number of appointments that a student must attend (NMC, 2019). The number of women in the case load that a student must complete, and the number of appointments a student must attend is determined by the individual university.

There may be a strategic choice of women for a student case load in order that workload is reduced, making it easier to balance the competing demands of practice, academia, case load, and personal life (Sweet & Glover, 2013). Multiparous women may need to be seen less regularly than primiparas, those who have had a previous precipitate labour may labour quickly again and so provide students with a shorter on-call shift for labour care, and women already nearing term would reduce the number of appointments needed and the duration of the continuity of carer experience (Sweet & Glover, 2013). Engaging in the continuity of carer experience in a non-meaningful way whereby students do not conduct the majority, if not all, of the woman's appointments means the student-woman relationship may be merely superficial. Students may not be welcomed by women, particularly during labour, if they are simply fulfilling the course requirements rather than providing true continuity of carer, and some students have falsified documentation to meet course requirements (Gray et al., 2013; McLachlan et al., 2013; Sweet & Glover, 2013; McKellar et al., 2014).

While women reported feeling 'happy' being cared for by a student because they provided extra support, kindness and advocacy, they felt dissatisfied if the student was not fully engaged in their care or fully committed to the experience (Stulz et al., 2020). Lack of commitment undermines the underlying philosophy of continuity of carer, that of holistic woman-centred midwifery care, and the potential for continuity of carer to confer improved outcomes to women (Sweet & Glover, 2013). Furthermore, it also calls into question the student's motivation for and expectations of the experience. If the engagement with the women in the case load is minimal, what does the student expect to learn from either a personal or professional perspective, and what does the student expect the woman to gain from being part of the continuity of carer experience?

Prior to initiating the experience, it may be beneficial for the student to establish their own and the supervising midwife's expectations in order that these can be negotiated to begin with, for example the level of engagement with women. In addition, these expectations should also be discussed when gaining consent from women wishing to participate so that decision-making is fully informed, and consent is valid. If a woman is expecting to be seen by the student at every single appointment, then she may be disappointed and not feel valued if she only sees the student sporadically throughout her care.

The commitment to be on-call for labour care during the continuity of carer experience is misaligned with the largely ad hoc provision of labour care in the UK, thus students may not anticipate the level of commitment this requires. Furthermore, students are being asked to work in a way that often their supervising midwife is not. Many midwives do not work in continuity of carer teams and so they will not be asked to provide on-call labour care alongside the student (Lewis et al., 2013).

**Box 6.6 Activity 6.4**

- What do you think women might expect from you in terms of your commitment to them and their care?
- What effect do you think these expectations might have on you; do you think they are realistic? How can you manage these?
- What might the impact on a woman be if you join the case load towards the end of her pregnancy?

## Human factors

Undertaking the continuity of carer experience is not without its challenges, yet it is these challenges as well as the rewards that prepare students for initiation of first post and future professional practice (Rawnson et al., 2013). Interweaving continuity of carer into the curriculum facilitates students to prepare for the experience, particularly if peer support is available so that students can learn from others who have recently completed the experience (Rawnson et al., 2013; McKellar et al., 2014). Similarly, students are expected to access support and supervision from a variety of sources, including practice and academic supervisors, and Professional Midwifery Advocates (Homer et al., 2008; Rawnson et al., 2013). This support network provides a safe space for reflection and re-engagement with the student's core values and the philosophy of woman-centred care that is central to continuity of carer (Rawnson et al., 2013).

Supervision by a community midwife with whom the student has already worked increases student confidence and preparedness for continuity of carer, optimises the learning potential of the experience, and makes students feel more supported (Rawnson et al., 2009). Regular reviews with the midwife supervising the experience contributes to safe practice and timely and effective feedback (Rawnson et al., 2009). Midwives who work in continuity of carer models report that the small teams in which they work are sources of support and provide opportunities for coaching between senior and more junior members, in turn leading to quicker consolidation of skills and development of confidence (Cummins et al., 2017). Furthermore, the opportunity to be supported by a small team enables midwives to reflect on practice and provides emotional support (Cummins et al., 2017), and it may be beneficial to replicate this during the continuity of carer experience in order to facilitate reflection and improve support.

A potential drawback of building close relationships in midwifery care is that practitioner's risk being exposed to the stress and trauma experienced by some of the women in their care, which may cause vicarious traumatisation of midwives and students alike (Homer et al., 2008). Participation in the emotional journeys of women may be challenging for students, and it needs to be considered how students are going to manage the emotional work of continuity of carer, and how they can reconcile this with other personal, academic and course obligations (Rawnson et al., 2011). There is, however, a paucity of literature pertaining to the emotional impact of continuity of carer on students.

While it is noted that the midwife-woman relationship is a source of emotion work in midwifery, a further source is that of the conflicting ideologies between community and hospital-based midwifery (Hunter, 2004). Novice practitioners such as student and newly qualified midwives are particularly vulnerable to this conflict due to their strongly held allegiance to holistic woman-centred care, which is in opposition to the medicalised philosophy of care that prevails in hospital-based midwifery (Hunter, 2004). Students may work across both community and hospital settings during the continuity of carer experience and may feel the strain of advocating for women in a model of care that requires them to affiliate with the institution rather than the woman. Women feel that students protect woman-centred care and values, and empower them (Stulz et al., 2020).

The continuity of carer experience is an opportunity for students to apply their academic learning to authentic real-world midwifery and to take ownership of that learning, in part by researching specific points of practice to inform and facilitate evidence-based decision-making with women (Rawnson et al., 2009). The experience is multifaceted and as well as learning how to be a midwife, it can teach students to integrate being a midwife into their daily lives, and to develop strategies to do this. Emotional intelligence, self-awareness and resilience are required to ensure the sustainability of continuity of carer (Homer et al., 2008) and, arguably, the sustainability of the midwifery workforce, regardless of the model of care in which midwives work. Self-awareness enables midwives and students to examine their own behaviours and attitudes and adjust them accordingly, in turn assisting them to cope with complex workloads (Homer et al., 2008).

---

**Box 6.7 Activity 6.5**

- What personal and professional rewards do you expect to gain from your case load?
- Who is your support network, what can they help you with, how can they support you?
- How are you going to reflect on and in practice, and do you feel comfortable reflecting with the supervising midwife?
- Think of a time that you have been affected emotionally by a woman's story or experience during your training. What effect did this have on you, how did you cope with or manage your emotions?

---

## Resilience and burnout

Becoming and being a midwife is a significant source of emotion work, which has been attributed to three factors: discrepancies between the idealised midwifery that students and midwives aspire to and the realities of practice; being with women in times of intense emotion and performing intimate care and procedures; feeling disenfranchised due to conflicts with managers who do not protect midwives' interests or well-being (Rayment, 2015). There exists an interrelation between high levels of burnout and poorer quality of care, low job satisfaction, and staff resignation (Stimpfel et al., 2012; Henriksen & Lukasse, 2016; Stoll & Gallagher, 2019), hence it is important for you to be able to mitigate against burnout. Seminal work exploring emotional labour at work found that being able to 'perform' certain emotions was an integral part of some professional roles (Hochschild, 1983). Workers were expected to display emotions appropriate to the situation to reassure clients, for example being calm and in control in emergency situations when the employee's natural reaction may otherwise have been one of fear or stress (Hochschild, 1983). Managing the outward display of emotions may be emotionally challenging, and the feelings shown should be adequate to demonstrate that midwives are human but should not invert the caring relationship such that families must care for a midwife who is significantly upset or distressed (Rayment, 2015). Part of the challenge of becoming a midwife is learning how to manage the emotional aspects (Figure 6.1) of the role so that they can continue to provide optimal woman-centred care in such an emotive environment, which may be especially challenging for novice practitioners who are yet to develop these skills (Rayment, 2015).

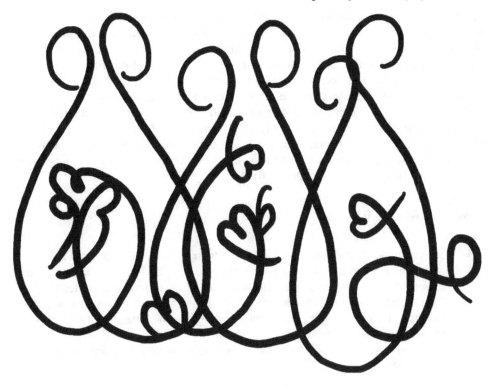

*Figure 6.1* Struggling with mixed emotions by Ashforth

The demands of a caring profession may be compounded by the expectation of self-sacrifice whereby midwives work through breaks and beyond contracted hours to finish their work or provide care for women, and by long shifts and inadequate staffing (Dent, 2019; RCM, 2019). Work-related stress may cause up to half of midwives to feel unwell, and the negative working practices are associated with increased absenteeism due to sickness, high levels of staff turnover, and higher rates of burnout (World Health Organisation (WHO), 2018). Burnout is a result of workplace stress that has not been well-managed, and is characterised by exhaustion, decreased efficacy at work, and feelings of negativity, cynicism or mental distance from one's job (WHO, 2018). While such organisational interventions as shorter shift lengths and shift patterns more conducive to a positive work-life balance may help to alleviate stress and thus burnout, these should be combined with personal interventions such as counselling or self-care (Dent, 2019).

Students and midwives alike need to learn strategies to manage workplace stress and the emotion work of midwifery to remain passionate and effective members of the workforce. Part of this learning needs to include resilience, described as the ability to bounce back from challenging, stressful or emotive experiences, which is key to well-being (Parry, 2017). In caring roles, resilience has been linked to acceptance, account-ability, empathy and empathic warmth (Parry, 2017). Acceptance relies on the ability to feel and acknowledge the emotions of others, accountability is the ability to be accountable to one's own reactions to those emotions, empathy requires experiences to be seen from the other person's perspective, and empathic warmth is the ability to care for the well-being of another (Parry, 2017). While it is a privilege to be part of a woman's childbirth journey, it can also be emotionally challenging and draining, yet as professionals, midwives can 'provide empathic warmth because of our ability to experience empathy safely and professionally' (Parry, 2017, p. 14). Students and midwives need to be able to recognise emotions and empathise with them, but without absorbing them or wearing those emotions themselves. Maintaining a safe distance from these emotions, keeping the professional and personal separate, and taking stock after particularly emotive situations may be crucial in developing resilience and safeguarding one's own well-being, which may be facilitated through engagement with clinical supervision, support from midwives, peers, family and friends, and writing reflective accounts (Parry, 2017; Dent, 2019).

---

**Box 6.8 Activity 6.6**

- Can you think of an experience during your training that you have found particularly emotional? What happened, how did you feel, and did you think it was appropriate for you to display emotions in front of the woman in this situation?
- Do you think it is possible to maintain a safe distance from the emotional work of midwifery, how might you achieve this, and do you think this might impact the way you practise as a midwife?
- Do you think you are resilient? Why/why not? How might you be able to improve your resilience?

---

## The future

Continuity of carer is expounded to be the future of maternity care due to improved outcomes for women, and job satisfaction for midwives (NMC, 2015; NHS England, 2017; Corrigan, 2017). As such, midwifery education must prepare a future workforce competent, confident and willing to provide continuity of carer in order to implement service changes that will improve rates of continuity of carer (Gamble et al., 2020). The case load held experience prepares students to work in continuity of carer models upon qualification (Cummins et al., 2017), and the experience needs to be built into a relevant academic module to highlight its importance within training and practice itself, with a focus on bridging the gap and placing woman-centred continuity of carer at the heart of both academic learning and practice placements (Gamble et al., 2020).

Continuity of carer teams of midwives have been demonstrated to confer such benefits as a shared philosophy of care, good working relationships, and open communication, and midwives working in a continuity of carer model have reported higher levels of job satisfaction than those working in standard models of care (Halse, 2019). Furthermore, the opportunities to reflect, debrief, and learn are more abundant in continuity of carer models, which may contribute to increased resilience in these midwives, and may mitigate against the challenges of continuity of carer and protect midwives against burnout. To mimic the positive aspects of continuity of carer models of care and to better replicate the experiences of continuity of carer, it could be considered that student group practices, or small case load teams should be established to provide continuity of carer to women.

This would give students the opportunity to experience continuity of carer more authentically than at present as case loading as an individual midwife or student midwife may be unrealistic. In this model, small groups of students could work collaboratively to provide continuity of carer, with women having a named student and a buddy student caring for them. The women would still receive continuity of carer and would know a second member of the team who could be on-call in case of a long labour and shift change. Students could handover care to the buddy student without feeling that the woman were missing out on continuity of carer. Students may enjoy the benefits of peer support for reflection and debriefing, which would provide extensive opportunities for learning and continued professional development.

---

**Box 6.9  Activity 6.7**

- Do you think that student group case-loading would be a realistic and authentic way of case-loading?
- What are the advantages and disadvantages to you as students and to the women?
- Might this be a realistic service improvement project for your university/Trust? What are the barriers to this?

---

**Box 6.10  Vignette 6.3: The midwife voice**

The continuity of carer experience is a demonstration of the student's skills, attributes, identity and professionalism, and while certain skills clusters must be achieved prior to qualification, each student and midwife will bring their own qualities and nuances to practice. This is an opportunity for students to showcase themselves as the midwives they are becoming. This includes care that is woman-centred, holistic, and individualised, not only to the woman but to the student. Across their training, students begin to incorporate various practices and aspects of care that they have seen demonstrated by midwives with whom they have worked. Continuity of carer enables students to tailor care according to their own philosophy and personality and should empower students to provide care in ways that are unique to them and the women in their case load. As midwives, it is our role to give students the freedom and confidence to do this, while maintaining safe, evidence-based, professional practice.

The pillars of professional practice are documented in the Code to which midwives and students must adhere (NMC, 2015) and, as with midwifery, this experience must reiterate the fact that as individuals we represent the profession as a collective, and that we have a commitment to and duty of care for women. As midwives, it is our responsibility to role model this so that core values and high standards of care are transferred to students and are subsequently demonstrated throughout their own practice.

These core values and philosophies are not only key to maintaining high quality holistic care, but also to developing the resilience necessary to face professional challenges that may arise. As midwives, we want to witness students honing their skills, including clinical reasoning and decision-making, and we acknowledge our part in this process. We also want students to take ownership of their case load and invest emotionally in it, meaning they feel a real sense of pride and achievement upon its completion. We remember how we felt as students undertaking continuity of carer. The feeling of humility and privilege that we were being invited to take part in a woman's story, the sense of purpose and longevity, the notion that each journey is individual to each woman, the realisation that being with woman (in whatever capacity is appropriate for her) can be enough. The ability to intuit the needs of the woman when no words are spoken, the intangible learning that goes beyond skill acquisition and box-ticking. The dedication to a case load that is inherent and is present not because it is mandated by the course, but because the student wants to be there for their own development and, more importantly, for the woman. We want students to want to be present every step of the way, and we believe that the learning objectives for the continuity of carer experience should remain true to the holistic nature of it. The achievement of learning objectives should be reviewed and revised at various points across the experience to ensure objectives are being met and remain relevant to practice. Similarly, reflection is an integral part of midwifery practice and must likewise form a key component of continuity of carer (see resources section for reflective model adapted from Ashforth, 2020).

---

**Box 6.11  Activity 6.8**

At the end of your case load, consider and reflect on the emotional journey of the experience. How did you feel at various stages of the case load? Now that the experience has ended, what have you learnt about the emotion work of being a midwife? How did you manage this aspect of midwifery?

---

## In summary

As presented, there are numerous things for you to consider when undertaking any aspect of midwifery care, but you may need to consider these aspects in a different way when undertaking a continuity of carer approach to care. You may have concluded that providing care in a continuity approach has benefits to not just the women, their families and the service, but to you as well. Your personal values and belief systems will support your thinking and development of resilience in the current health care systems. Remind yourself what brought you to the world of midwifery and if this reality was what you expected it to be like. If it is different, what makes it different and what do you need to reconsider to ensure your focus remains as you wish it to be. The following chapter may help you with this activity.

## References

Allen, J., Kildea, S., Hartz, D., Tracy, M., & Tracy, S. (2017). The motivation and capacity to go 'above and beyond'. Qualitative analysis of free-text survey responses in the M@NGO randomised controlled trial of case load midwifery. *Midwifery*, 50: 148–156.
Ashforth, K. (2020). Exploring the woman-student-midwife relationship: a critical relationship on practice. *The Student Midwife*, 3(2). Available at: www.all4maternity.com/exploring-th

e-woman-student-midwife-relationship-a-critical-reflection-on-practice/ [accessed: 13 September, 2020].

Ashforth, K., & Kitson-Reynolds, E. (2019a). Fairy tale midwifery ten years on: Re-evaluating the lived experiences of newly qualified midwives. *British Journal of Midwifery*, 27(10): 649–654. Available at: www.magonlinelibrary.com/doi/full/10.12968/bjom.2 019.27.10.649.

Ashforth, K., & Kitson-Reynolds, E. (2019b). Fairy tale midwifery ten years on: Facilitating the transition to newly qualified midwife. *BJOM*, 27(122): 782–789.

Aune, I., Dahlberg, U., & Ingebrigsten, O. (2011). Relational continuity as a model of care in practical midwifery studies. *BJOM*, 19(8): 515–523.

Blomberg, K., & Sahlberg-Blom, E. (2007). Closeness and distance: A way of handling difficult situation. *Journal of Clinical Nursing*, 16: 244–254.

Browne, J., Haora, P.J., Taylor, J., & Davis, D.L. (2014). 'Continuity of care' experiences in midwifery education: Perspectives from diverse stakeholders. *Nurse Education in Practice*, 14(5): 573–578.

Collins, C., Fereday, J., Pincombe, J., Oster, C., & Turnbull, D. (2010). An evaluation of the satisfaction of midwives working in midwifery group practice. *Midwifery*, 26(4): 435–441.

Corrigan, A. (2017). Continuity of carer and application of the Code: How student midwives can be agents of change. *British Journal of Midwifery*, 25(8).

Cummins, A.M., Catling, C., & Homer, C.S.E. (2017). Enabling new graduate midwives to work in continuity of carer models: A conceptual model for implementation. *Women and Birth*, 31(5): 343–349.

Dawson, K., Newton, M., Forster, D., & McLachlan, H. (2018). Comparing case load and non-case load midwives' burnout levels and professional attitudes: A national, cross-sectional survey of Australian midwives working in the public maternity system. *Midwifery*, 63: 60–67.

Dent, J. (2019). In the line of duty: The emotional wellbeing of midwives. *The Practising Midwife*, 22: 8. Available at: www.all4maternity.com/in-the-line-of-duty-the-emotional-well being-of-midwives/ [accessed: 9 September, 2020].

Fenwick, J., Toohill, J., Slavin, V., et al. (2018). Improving psychoeducation for women fearful of childbirth: Evaluation of a research translation project. *Women and Birth*, 31(1): 1–9.

Fereday, J., & Oster, C. (2010). Managing a work–life balance: The experiences of midwives working in a group practice setting. *Midwifery*, 26: 311–318.

Fry, J., Rawnson, S., & Lewis, P. (2013). Problems and practicalities in student case load holding. *British Journal of Midwifery*, 19(10).

Gamble, J., Sidebotham, M., Gilkison, A., Davis, D., & Sweet, L. (2020). Acknowledging the primacy of continuity of care experiences in midwifery education. *Women and Birth*, 33(2): 111–118.

Gilkison, A., McAra-Couper, J., Gunn, J., Crowther, S., Hunter, M., Macgregor, D., & Hotchin, C. (2010). Midwifery practice arrangements which sustain case loading: Lead Maternity Care midwives in New Zealand. *New Zealand College of Midwives Journal*, 51: 11–16.

Gray, J., Leap, N., Sheehy, A., & Homer, C. (2013). Students' perceptions of the follow-through experience in three year bachelor of midwifery programme in Australia. *Midwifery*, 29(4): 400–406.

Halse, A.-M. (2019). A reflection on a philosophy of care All4maternity. *The Student Midwife Journal*, 2(1).

Henriksen, L., & Lukasse, M. (2016). Burnout among Norwegian midwives and the contribution of personal and work-related factors: A cross-sectional study. *Sex Reprod Health*, 9: 42–47.

Hochschild, A. (1983). *The Managed Heart: Commercialisation of Human Feeling*. Berkeley: University of California Press.

Homer, C., Leap, N., & Brodie, P. (2008). *Midwifery Continuity of Care: A Practical Guide*. Sydney: Elsevier.

Hughes, A., & Fraser, D. (2011). 'There are guiding hands and there are controlling hands': Student midwives' experiences of mentorship in the UK. *Midwifery*, 27(6): 786–792.

Hunter, B. (2004). Conflicting ideologies as a source of emotion work in midwifery. *Midwifery*, 20(3): 261–272.

Jefford, E., Nolan, S.J., Sansone, H., et al. (2020). 'A match made in midwifery': Women's perceptions of student midwife partnerships. *Women and Birth*, 33(2): 193–198.

Kramer, M. (1974). Reality shock: Why nurses leave nursing California. The CV Mosby Company.

Lewis, P., Fry, J., & Rawnson, S. (2013). Student midwife case-loading: A new approach to midwifery education. *British Journal of Midwifery*, 16(8).

McKellar, L., Charlick, S., Warland, J., & Birbeck, D. (2014). Access, boundaries and confidence: The ABC of facilitating continuity of care experience in midwifery education. *Women and Birth*, 27: 61–66.

McLachlan, H., Newton, M., Nightingale, H., Morrow, J., & Kruger, G. (2013). Exploring the follow-through experience: A state-wide survey of midwifery students and academics conducted in Victoria Australia. *Midwifery*, 29(9): 1064–1072.

Moncrieff, G., MacVicar, S., Norris, G., & Hollins Martin, C. (2020). Optimising the continuity experiences of student midwives: An integrative review. *Women and Birth*. Available at: https://doi.org/10.1016/j.wombi.2020.01.007 [accessed: 28 December, 2020].

National Institute for Health and Care Excellence (2019). Antenatal care for uncomplicated pregnancies. Clinical Guidance CG62. Available at: www.nice.org.uk/guidance/cg62/chapter/1-Guidance#clinical-examination-of-pregnant-women [accessed: 7 September, 2020].

NHS England (2017). Implementing better births: Continuity of carer. Available at www.england.nhs.uk/publication/implementingbetter-births-continuity-of-carer [accessed: 29 November, 2020].

Nursing and Midwifery Council (2010). *The MiNT Project*. London: NMC. Available at: www.nmc.org.uk/globalassets/siteDocuments/Midwifery-Reports/MINT-report.pdf [accessed: 1 September, 2020].

Nursing and Midwifery Council (2015/2018). *The Code: Standards of Conduct, Performance and Ethics for Nurses and Midwives*. London: NMC.

Nursing and Midwifery Council (2019). *Realising Professionalism: Standards for Education and Training*. London: NMC. Available at: www.nmc.org.uk/globalassets/sitedocuments/education-standards/education-framework.pdf [accessed: 1 September, 2020].

Parry, S. (2017). Preface: Sharing stories as a means of exploring experiences. In S. Parry (Ed.), *Effective Self-Care and Resilience in Clinical Practice*. London: Jessica Kingsley Publishers.

Pugh, J.D., Twigg, D.E., Martin, T.L., & Rai, T. (2013). Western Australia facing critical losses in its midwifery workforce: A survey of midwives' intentions. *Midwifery*, 29: 497–505.

Rawnson, S., Brown, S., Wilkins, C., & Leamon, J. (2009). Student midwives' views of case loading: The BUMP study. *British Journal of Midwifery*, 17(8). doi:10.12968/bjom.2009.17.8.43640.

Rawnson, S. (2011). A qualitative study exploring student midwives' experiences of carrying a case load as part of their midwifery education in England. *Midwifery*, 2(6), 786–792.

Rayment, J. (2015). Emotional labour: How midwives manage emotions at work. *The Practising Midwife*. Available at: www.all4maternity.com/emotional-labour-midwives-manage-emotion-work/ [accessed: 9 September, 2020].

Royal College of Midwives (2019). England short of almost 2500 midwives, new birth figures confirm. Available at: www.rcm.org.uk/news-views/rcm-opinion/2019/england-short-of-almost-2-500-midwives-new-birth-figures-confirm/ [accessed: 19 September, 2020].

Sidebotham, M., & Fenwick, J. (2019). Midwifery students' experiences of working within a midwifery case load model. *Midwifery*, 74, 21–28.

Siebold, C. (2015). The experiences of a first cohort of Bachelor of Midwifery students Victoria, Australia. *Austr Midwifery J*, 18(3): 9–16.

Stimpfel, A.W., Sloane, D.M., & Aiken, L.H. (2012). The longer the shifts for hospital nurses, the higher the levels of burnout and patient dissatisfaction. *Healt Aff*, 31(11): 2501–2509.

Stoll, K., & Gallagher, J. (2019). A survey of burnout and intentions to leave the profession among Western Canadian midwives. *Women and Birth*, 32(4): e441–e449.

Stulz, V., Elmir, R., & Reilly, H. (2020). Evaluation of a student-led midwifery group practice: A woman's perspective. *Midwifery*, 86.

Styles, C., Kearney, L., & George, K. (2020). Implementation and upscaling of midwifery continuity of care: The experience of midwives and obstetricians. *Women and Birth*, 33(4): 343–351.

Sullivan, K., Lock, L., & Homer, C.S.E. (2011). Factors that contribute to midwives staying in midwifery: A study in one area health service in New South Wales, Australia. *Midwifery*, 27: 331–335.

Sweet, L.P., & Glover, P. (2013). An exploration of the midwifery continuity of care program at one Australian university as a symbiotic clinical education model. *Nurse Education Today*, 33: 262–267.

Wentworth, I. (2020). What midwives think of the continuity of carer model. *British Journal of Midwifery* 28(7): 403–405.

WHO (2018). *International Classification of Diseases*, 11th revision (ICD-11). Geneva: WHO.

Zapf, D. (2002). Emotion work and psychological well-being: A review of the literature and some conceptual considerations. *Human Resourcing Management Review* 12: 237–268.

# 7 Case load held experience lifelong learning and professional development

*Emer Kelly, Kate Ashforth, Ellen Kitson-Reynolds and Lesley Turner*

## Introduction

The role of the student and qualified midwife encompasses that of public health to reduce health inequalities and optimise outcomes for women and their families. To provide a service and workforce that are responsive to current and ever-changing healthcare complexities, midwifery education and training must be adaptable and engage students in research-based modules that focus on evidence-based practice. Development of criticality will give both you and midwives alike, the skills to assess evidence and provide care that is relevant and based on high-quality evidence. Continued professional development and reflection on and in practice are required to maintain professional registration and to ensure that care is compassionate and woman centred. Professional development also requires students and midwives to access sources of support, including professional midwifery advocates, which may mitigate against work-related stress and burnout, in turn reducing absenteeism and attrition rates.

> **Box 7.1 Activity 7.1**
>
> Consider your own learning style.
>
> - How do you best learn?
> - Do you need to be with others?
> - What benefits to your own learning are there when in groups and when on your own?
> - What motivates you to learn and complete tasks?
> - Do you have self-determination and self-discipline when it comes to learning and updating your knowledge and skills?

## Curriculum development

Midwifery education, and how it can and should prepare midwives of the future, was an integral part of Midwifery 2020 (CNO, 2010). While the document is chronologically outdated, its ideas are still pertinent: the future of midwifery depends on a workforce that is competent, accountable, and autonomous at the point of registration. A complex and rapidly changing healthcare environment means it is crucial that

DOI: 10.4324/9781003051527-7

*Table 7.1* Standards for education and training

| Part | Element |
| --- | --- |
| One | Standards framework for nursing and midwifery (NMC, 2018a) |
| Two | Standards for student supervision and assessment (NMC, 2018b) |
| Three | Standards for pre-registration midwifery programmes (NMC, 2019) |

the best available evidence informs not only midwifery practice but also midwifery education, both of which must be responsive and relevant to such changes.

As such, the Nursing and Midwifery Council (NMC) (2018a; 2018b; 2019) have recently published their new Standards for Education and Training, summarised in Table 7.1.

UK-based higher and approved education institutions (AEIs) should be working towards a midwifery curriculum that reflect these new standards, as well as the changing world of midwifery both nationally and internationally (WHO, 2019). Timely feedback from service-users and colleagues is essential to enhance learning through real-world practice-based placements (Haycock-Stuart et al., 2016). Programmes may also wish to incorporate Renfrew et al.'s (2014) framework for quality maternal and newborn care, the principles of the 6 Cs (Cummings & Bennet, 2012), Better Births (The National Maternity Review, 2016), the NHS 5-year plan (2019), The Lancet series for midwifery (Renfrew et al., 2014) and the International Confederation of Midwives (ICM) (2017; 2019) definition of a midwife.

## Evidence-based practice

While it is understood that midwives must 'always practise in line with the best available evidence' (NMC, 2015), evidence itself has its own strengths and limitations:

> Evidence-based practice (EBP) … involves complex and conscientious decision-making based not only on the available evidence but also on patient characteristic, situations and preferences.
>
> (McKibbon, 1998, p. 399)

Midwifery education should therefore embed knowledge of research methods within its curriculum, enabling students to apply research to practice. Modules teaching students to analyse and critique an array of research should lead to a sense of criticality essential to evaluating evidence and providing true EBP. High-quality research is vital to support changes and developments in midwifery practices and improve experiences for women, thus as a student you need to recognise and appreciate this fundamental role of the midwife and acknowledge that this continues when qualified. At the point of registration, regardless of where you trained and what pathway you took to becoming a qualified midwife, you must be able to demonstrate the professional qualities, skills, knowledge and behaviours expected of a new registrant, including EBP.

## Public health role

Moving forwards with policy commitments to reducing health inequalities in the UK and the focus on optimising health and preventing disease, midwives must further enhance their public health role (Department of Health (DH) et al., n.d.). As both a student and qualified midwife, you play a key role in assessing the health and social needs and delivering the public health agenda. An example of this is the midwife's role in perinatal mental health. Maternal mental health is crucial not only in improving women's well-being, but also in protecting and optimising the health of the woman's whole support network, including that of the newborn (Phelan, 2010; The Nuffield Trust, 2017). Babies born to women who have undiagnosed and unmanaged mental health concerns are at an increased risk of adverse outcomes; these include poor bonding and attachment (Muzik & Borovska, 2010; Hoffman et al., 2017). Women at risk of poor quality of life, self-harm, and suicide, with mental health conditions cited as cause of death for 10% of maternal deaths in 2015–2017 (MBRRACE-UK, 2019). It is acknowledged that while 'most' women should receive continuity of carer by 2021, '75% of women from BAME [Black, Asian and Minority Ethnic] communities and a similar percentage of women from the most deprived groups will receive continuity of care' (NHS England, 2019, p. 41). The focus on women from 'BAME'/ 'Black and Brown'/'Black and Asian' communities and deprived areas aims to address stark inequalities in neonatal and maternal morbidity and mortality: women in these groups are more likely to experience a stillbirth or neonatal death and are up to five times more likely to die during pregnancy and the puerperium (MBRRACE-UK 2019; 2020a; 2020b). While it is anticipated that continuity of carer will improve outcomes and reduce health inequalities, extending continuity of carer has been, and will continue to be, a complex task that includes a risk management perspective, driven by rules and protocols that overlook individual needs and circumstances (Bryar & Sinclair, 2011).

## Practice supervision and assessment

The NMC standards for education and training replace the Standards for Learning and Assessment in Practice (SLAiP) (NMC, 2008) and the role of the mentor and sign-off mentor, by introducing a practice supervisor, practice assessor and academic assessor (NMC, 2018b) mode of support and assessment (see also Chapters 4 and 5). Despite a move away from the 1:1 mentor support and assessment requirements (Health Education England, 2018) previously set out, the new standards for nursing and midwifery education state that practice will continue to be assessed to determine progress and competence (NMC, 2018a; 2018b; 2018c; 2018d). The NMC Standards for student supervision and assessment (SSSA) set out expectations for the learning, support and supervision of students in the practice environment (NMC, 2018). The key principles are:

- Effective practice learning – All students are provided with safe, effective and inclusive learning experiences.
- Supervision of students – Practice supervision enables students to learn and safely achieve proficiency and autonomy in their professional role.
- Assessment of students and confirmation of proficiency – Student assessments are evidence-based, robust and objective.

The role of the practice assessor is to conduct and record objective, fair, evidenced-based assessments. For this to happen, each practice supervisor must clearly document and provide evidence demonstrating the student's progress (NMC, 2018b). NMC registered nurses and midwives as well as other registered health and social care professionals may supervise nursing and midwifery students in the role of practice supervisor. The practice supervisor will 'support and supervise students, providing feedback on their progress towards and achievement of proficiencies and skills' (NMC, 2018: 3.3). The practice assessor will 'conduct assessments to confirm student achievement of proficiencies and programme outcomes for practice learning', and 'assessment decisions by practice assessors are informed by feedback sought and received from practice supervisors' (NMC, 2018: 7.1 and 7.2). All students will be assigned a different academic assessor for each part of the education programme' (NMC, 2018: 6.1) and, while the practice supervisor does not have to be a midwife, the practice assessor does. A midwife can be both a practice supervisor and a practice assessor but cannot be both simultaneously for the same student to reduce the risk of bias. The coherent and standardised approach to supervising and assessing students in practice aims to ensure the safety of women, babies and their families whilst supporting students to develop as midwives.

Grading in practice had been integrated within the NMC midwifery education standards since 2009 in order that equal emphasis was placed on practice and theory (NMC, 2009). Practice, direct hands-on care, remains a requirement of midwifery education programmes and must contribute to a minimum of fifty per cent of midwifery training programmes (and a minimum of 2300 hours (NMC, 2019)), although does not specify the proportion of attributed credits, if any, aligning with the World Health Organisation (WHO, 2009) requirement of a balance between theory and practice components. Assessment within practice is well documented (Heaslip & Scammell, 2012) and grading in practice is not without its challenges and can be open to subjectiveness, obscurity, inconsistency and grade inflation (Donaldson & Gray, 2012), although this should be mitigated against by the introduction of SSSA. The difficulty of ensuring consistency, reliability and validity in practice assessment tools and approaches is challenging (Fisher et al., 2011; Seldomridge et al., 2006; Dalton et al., 2009), and grading should focus on a student's performance during their period of 'practice supervision' (NMC, 2018b). Feedback from practice supervisors and service users is fundamental, and objective, evidence-based assessments must provide constructive feedback to facilitate professional development (NMC, 2018b, p. 10). Some AEIs are now implementing a form of grading for students to be able to assess their progress against throughout their programmed years, but this may not contribute to degree classifications overall. You, as a student undertaking this part of your curriculum' are introduced to the lifelong learning and continuous professional development within practice from the start of your midwifery journey continuing through your career as a midwife supporting the next generation of learners.

**Box 7.2 Activity 7.2**

Reflect on the strengths and limitations of your experience assessments in practice and consider how you will support future learners as both a student and a qualified midwife?

*Table 7.2* Evidence required for revalidation (NMC, 2016)

| Component of revalidation | Requirements |
| --- | --- |
| Practice Hours | • 450 hours. |
| CPD | • 35 hours, of which a minimum of 20 hours must be participatory.<br>• Give a description of the topic and how it related to your practice.<br>• How did it relate to the Code. |
| Practice-related feedback | • Five pieces of feedback.<br>• From service users, colleagues, managers.<br>• Can be verbal or written, formal or informal. |
| Written reflective accounts | • Five written reflections.<br>• Related to CPD and/or.<br>• Practice-related feedback and/or.<br>• An event or experience in practice. |
| Reflective discussion | • Undertaken with another NMC registrant.<br>• A discussion about your five reflective accounts.<br>• How do your reflections relate to the Code. |
| Health and character | • Declaration of health and character.<br>• Are there any impairments to your fitness to practice?<br>• Have you been subject to any cautions or criminal charges? |
| Professional indemnity arrangement | • Confirm that you have, or will have when practising, cover under an indemnity arrangement. |
| Confirmation | • A declaration by yourself and the NMC registrant confirming that the Revalidation process has been carried out and all components achieved. |

## Professional revalidation

To maintain their professional registration, midwives in the UK must revalidate every three years. Revalidation promotes good practice and enables midwives to demonstrate that they are practising safely and effectively (NMC, 2016). Revalidation is a demonstration of a midwife's fitness to practice and requires that the midwife submits evidence outlined in Table 7.2.

## Practice-based learning

Practice-based learning is essential in ensuring future midwives are fit for practice and purpose (NMC, 2015). An effective practice-based learning opportunity is one in which the intended competencies and learning outcomes are well-defined and understood by both educator/professional and student, and where roles and responsibilities of the AEI, placement area and you (the student) are equally clear (The Quality Assurance Agency, 2012). As a student, you will need to have your own realistic expectations and should understand the expectations of professionals with whom you are working, furthermore you should have a clear idea of what you need and want to achieve in each placement area.

Professionals have a responsibility to ensure that opportunities, resources and supervision are available so that learning outcomes can be met, which will enable students to work towards registration. Learning opportunities may depend on the professionals with whom you work, which is explored more extensively in Chapter 6, and the shift away from mentorship to practice supervision and assessment may mean you need to be more proactive in seeking out learning opportunities. A provisional allocation of a student to a practice supervisor at the start of each shift may mean that you are unlikely to work with the same person consistently, hence you will be responsible for ensuring you are meeting your own targets and developing your skills. While the aims of SSSA (NMC, 2018) is to minimise the risk of bias to student grading in practice, avoid the so-called failure to fail students, and better prepare the future workforce for the process of revalidation, it has been anecdotally suggested that students may feel less adequately supported when working with previously unknown midwives than with mentors. This may in turn inhibit student confidence and skill acquisition (Cook-Saher & Wilson, 2020). Similarly, students experienced an increased sense satisfaction and ease when on placement within a continuity of carer team and saw a more explicit woman-centred philosophy of care than when working in other placement settings (Gray et al., 2013; Dawson et al., 2015). The new standards for education state that all student midwives should experience continuity of carer throughout their training (NMC, 2019) which may in turn encourage midwives of the future to accept this as the new normal and mean more midwives are open to work in this way. A continuity of carer experience, whether as part of student case loading or as a placement within a continuity of carer team is believed to enhance student confidence and competence (Gilmour et al., 2013). This may be because the philosophy of care is more closely aligned to that of the student, or because the small teams mean that students feel well-supported to learn in a positive practice environment. Best practice values that within your future career as a midwife, you will be involved in continuous professional development directly in the practice setting and within an inter-professional team such as case reviews, audit and PROMPT training as examples (PROMPT Maternity Foundation, 2020). The NMC (2016) revalidation process ensures that continuous professional development contains both self-directed and 'in groups' activities across three years.

### Continued professional development

Continuous professional development plays a pivotal role to both students and qualified midwives. Values-based education (VBE) plays a role in the student midwife journey (Chapter 1), which encourages reflection and the maintenance of personal and professional values (Kitson-Reynolds, 2020). Once qualified, midwives are expected to engage in a range of continuous professional development activities to deliver safe, contemporary midwifery care that is responsive to developments in practice and service user requirements. Continuous professional development is also required to maintain professional registration with the NMC through the revalidation process, which will be discussed later in this chapter. While skill acquisition is pivotal for continuous professional development, some aspects of learning appear easier than others, for example learning to think critically is found to be more difficult than simply learning to perform a skill (Payan-Carreira et al., 2019). Furthermore, focusing on the doing or 'competence' of becoming a midwife is perceived to develop more easily for students than understanding the experience for the individual (Gilkison, Giddings, & Smythe, 2015). Similarly, some students struggle with reflecting on their experience.

Reflection on and in practice maximises learning both as students and as qualified midwives (Embo et al., 2015; Persson et al., 2015; Joyce-McCoach & Smith, 2016; Carter et al., 2017). Reflection is the thought process whereby individuals consider their experiences to gain insights about their whole practice, and it supports individuals to continually improve the way they work or the quality of care they give to people (Armstrong et al., 2017). Reflection should be a familiar, continuous element embedded into the work of all health care professionals and is a process that benefits midwives and the wider multidisciplinary team by discussing and exploring aspects of practice, building a collective understanding through discussion, knowledge and knowledge sharing (Wain et al., 2017). Collaborative working and learning increase the likelihood of affecting meaningful and positive change (Ghaye, 2007). Reflective practice is integral to continued registration through revalidation, continuing professional development, and continuing education requirements (Wain et al., 2017). It provides opportunity to evaluate our midwifery clinical practice experiences and apply current knowledge to gain new insight to inform and change our future practice (Bolton, 2014; Bass et al., 2017). Reflection assists with experiential learning and the development of critical thinking skills to bridge the theory-practice gap.

### Confidence and competence

The concepts of competence and confidence are not the same but may be linked. Confidence is defined as 'a feeling of self-assurance arising from an appreciation of one's own abilities or qualities'. Competence is defined as 'the ability to do something successfully or efficiently' (Oxford Dictionary, 2016).

Midwives need to have contact with women in a personal and professional way. With regards to the personal side, self-efficacy is required. Self-efficacy is described, as 'the belief in one's capabilities to organise and execute the courses of action required managing prospective situations' (Bandura, 1995, p. 2). Berggren (2003), when describing midwives' attitudes associated with the development of professional competence assumed this to grow with experience. Norman & Hyland (2003) identified that development of professional competence is dependent on circumstances relating to the workplace, and confidence can rise or fall. They meant that confidence can be linked to a sense of personal security and may be increased when a person feels secure and receives positive feedback (Norman & Hyland, 2003). This is evident within the midwifery literature which shows a need for a sense of belonging to the team (Gilmour et al., 2013). Therefore, staff who feel part of a team are more motivated, less anxious and display greater confidence (Levett-Jones & Lathlean, 2009), which seemingly supports findings that students working in continuity of carer teams feel similarly.

Increased levels of confidence may not be in proportion to increased competence, but decreased confidence could be linked to a decrease in skilled performance (Donovan, 2008). Confidence is of real importance to midwives especially in terms of patient safety, as well as other factors such as being able to communicate effectively with a woman in labour, establish a rapport and make her feel safe. Effective communication, having the right attitude and the need for the midwife to be inspired, caring, and kind are paramount (Butler et al., 2008; Byrom & Downe, 2010; Halldorsdottir & Karlsdottir, 2011; Thelin et al., 2014). An environment that offers a warm, supportive and friendly place to learn can strongly contribute towards enhancing competence and confidence. For students, clinical placement can be both physically and mentally challenging as events in pregnancy, labour and the postnatal period can quickly become very complex. Continuity of carer and case loading are fundamental in the provision of woman-centred care (McCourt et al., 2006). Caring for a case load of women gives students the opportunity to work closely with women and their families, developing trusting and worthwhile relationships, which in turn can enhance deeper learning and confidence. Anderson & Davies (2004) emphasise the importance of integrating cognitive and affective domains of learning in midwifery education, to ensure that the 'scientific' medicalised element of midwifery does not prevent the 'art' of midwifery. This is important to develop a sensitive approach to caring underpinning empathy and support which is evident with continuity of carer.

> **Box 7.3 Activity 7.3**
>
> Reflect on how you manage to provide quality care to women and their families when you feel under pressure, tired, out of your comfort zone due to limited knowledge and/or practical experience. Try to recall an event where you did not understand or know how to undertake a clinical aspect of care. How did you feel? How did it affect your ability to perform, communicate and focus? Once you learned and rehearsed this activity how did you feel and what impact did this have on your confidence to perform other aspects of care?

Student midwives' experience with case loading can enhance personal competence as well as confidence in developing skills and professional development, enabling evidenced-based practitioners on qualification. Exposure to the whole childbearing journey and working to full scope of practice has the potential to adapt midwives through personal and professional development, accountability, responsibility and reflective practice (NMC, 2019). According to The Better Birth's (NHS England, 2016) education has a key role to play in the preparation of the future workforce to enable them to accept working in continuity of care models when qualified. Research suggests newly qualified midwives have higher job satisfaction when working in continuity of carer models but have insufficient skills to initiate effective professional relationships with women and find it challenging to continue appropriate boundaries within the caring relationship (Cummins et al., 2015; 2017; Fereday & Oster, 2010). As Barrie (2004) considers, future midwives must have intellectual self-sufficiency, excellent communication and decision-making skills, and ethical and social understanding if they are to be employable and successful in their careers.

## Lifelong learning: starting with preceptorship

The preceptorship period provides the foundation for a lifelong journey of continuing professional development and reflective practice, as well as enabling midwives to develop a sense of self as they begin their career and prepare for revalidation. Preceptorship can be defined as:

A period of structured transition for the newly registered practitioner during which he or she will be supported by a preceptor, to develop their confidence as an autonomous professional, refine skills, values and behaviours and to continue on their journey of lifelong learning.

(DH, 2010)

It aims to provide support and guidance, enabling 'new registrants' to make the transition from student to accountable practitioner. This support provides guidance to practise in accordance with the professional code to which midwives must adhere (NMC, 2015). The reality of midwifery is that it can be emotionally, mentally and physically stressful and more and more midwives seek flexible ways of working in order to juggle both personal and professional demands. Attrition from the midwifery profession is increased in the first few years after qualification because midwives feel they cannot practise as they expected (Hughes & Fraser, 2011; Foster & Ashwin, 2014; RCM, 2017). In view of these factors, the Royal College of Midwives (RCM) conducted the 'Work Health and Emotional Lives of Midwives' (WHELM) study (Hunter et al., 2018) to provide stronger evidence about workforce wellbeing and the factors that influence this. The study found high levels of burnout, which were highest among younger midwives, those with less experience, and those working clinically, particularly within hospital and integrated settings. Workplace stress and feelings of burnout contribute to attrition amongst midwives; hence preceptorship is vital in supporting the transition from student to a confident and accountable midwife, which can be demanding and overwhelming (Ashforth & Kitson-Reynolds, 2019). Preceptorship supports newly qualified midwives through their transition by reducing stress and burnout, and increasing confidence and competence, while also building resilience, experience and professional accountability (DH, 2004; NMC, 2006; Hughes & Fraser, 2011; DH, 2015; Ashforth & Kitson-Reynolds, 2019).

## Continuous professional development: extended role of the midwife

Midwives engage in continuous professional development in a multitude of ways, not least by taking on extended roles within midwifery practice. Such specialist roles include practice education, perinatal mental health, case loading teams for vulnerable women, and fetal medicine midwives. Another such role pertains to the newborn infant physical examination (NIPE), also called examination of the newborn (EXON). Until 1996, NIPE was performed by paediatricians in hospital and general practitioners in community settings (Clarke & Simms, 2012). Practice subsequently changed to allow specially trained midwives to undertake NIPE, the justifications for which were continuity of carer, increasing autonomous practice and reducing doctors' working hours (Mitchell & Davies, 2016; Ashforth, 2020). Numerous AEIs provide NIPE training as part of their pre-registration midwifery training, which may further enhance continuity as students would be able to participate in NIPE for their case load. In terms of continuity once qualified, a greater number of midwives being NIPE-trained may enhance continuity as midwives working in continuity of carer teams would be able to also perform NIPE. For those in non-continuity models of care this may not be the case as NIPE would be performed by whichever midwife is on shift.

## Clinical supervision

Midwives benefit from supportive supervision which would enable safe, open conversations and opportunity to reflect upon potential challenges they may face in practice (Brodie, 2013). Restorative Clinical Supervision (RCS) addresses the emotional needs of staff and supports the development of resilience, enabling a 'thinking' space through discussion and reflective conversation, with open and honest feedback (Pettit & Stephen, 2015; NHS England, 2017). RCS assists midwives with their practice and works towards supporting clear thinking and decision-making through a process of reflection, so that stress and anxiety relating to work-related issues can be alleviated (Wallbank & Woods, 2012). Research suggests that the benefits of this positively impacts emotional wellbeing, reducing levels of stress and anxiety which in turn may reduce levels of sickness and staff leaving the profession (Wallbank & Woods, 2012).

The need for RCS is heightened due to the pressures experienced by the midwifery workforce in the face of the current Covid-19 pandemic. RCS could be incorporated within mandatory training to allow for an annual update, although midwives may need more regular RCS for it to be effective and some may feel reluctant to discuss sensitive issues in an open group setting. Challenges to supervision include staffing shortages, acuity onwards, cancellation of study days and CPD activities due to the pandemic and social distancing measures. Midwives may also feel reluctant to discuss sensitive issues in an open group.

A new model of midwifery supervision was developed in the UK based on recommendations of the 'Midwifery supervision and regulations: recommendations for change' (PHSO, 2013) and 'Midwifery regulation in the United Kingdom' (Baird et al., 2015). This resulted in the 'A-EQUIP' model of midwifery supervision (NHS England, 2017), which integrated three key elements – Restorative clinical supervision, Quality improvement and Education and development. The development of A-EQUIP and the associated role of the Professional Midwifery Advocate (PMA) have been devised in association with maternity service users, midwives, academics, midwifery and nurse leaders and managers, commissioners, the Royal College of Midwives (RCM) and Birth rights. PMAs are experienced practising midwives who have undergone extra training to support and guide midwives to deliver high quality and safe care. Each student and qualified midwife should choose a PMA that is going to support them in practice, for example in statement writing, reflection and debriefing, and with Revalidation, and the role is now confined to a supportive and advocacy function, rather than an investigatory one as was the case with the now defunct Supervisor of Midwife role.

### Box 7.4 Vignette 7.1: Reflection on practice

PMA: Tell me about the experience you want to share with me.
MIDWIFE: I have been caring for a woman who is G3 P1+1. This pregnancy follows a still birth at term. I provided all of the antenatal and postnatal care for her pregnancy with her second child, and was unable to find the baby's heartbeat at the term appointment. She is now 24 weeks' pregnant in her third pregnancy.
PMA: How do you feel about that – caring for her again?

MIDWIFE: I am terrified and feel a huge sense of pressure to get the care right and to provide care that is compassionate and holistic for her and her family, and to protect myself which is difficult.

PMA: What do you mean?

MIDWIFE: I want to tell her it is ok. I want to tell her that it's very unlikely that she'll leave hospital without a live baby this time, but for her she's had one good and one bad outcome so it's 50/50 whether this pregnancy will end well in her mind. There is always an automatic need to reassure people. I want to say I am sure it will be fine, but I cannot tell her that. I am sure it will be ok, but I cannot say that because there are no guarantees, and she knows that. It is interesting - me and the woman have been through an incredibly emotional journey together, and my priority has been her, quite rightly. At the same time, she was worrying about me, she seemed to know that I would be scared and was trying to reassure me as much as I was trying to reassure her. We both fear that we are going to listen in and I am not going to find a heartbeat again.

PMA: Did you ever debrief after this event with the woman and/or with a professional?

MIDWIFE: I did all her postnatal care. I saw her maybe 4–5 times at home. We all debriefed together, the husband, woman, and me. I am not sure it was what I needed, but they needed it, or maybe it was what I needed. I think it is difficult to talk to colleagues about this sometimes because as soon as you talk to someone they are quick to jump in and try to 'fix it' saying 'oh something similar happened to me'. They are trying to be empathetic, but it almost brushes it aside for you.

PMA: What happens to your practice because of this …

MIDWIFE: It impacts on the whole of my practice. If a woman comes in and says to you, I have not felt my baby move today or that the baby's movements have completely changed. I have 'fear and anxiety' that I am going to have to have this conversation with someone again. Fear of you having to say to someone that I cannot find your baby's heartbeat and they look to you for immediate answers, but you cannot diagnose this. You cannot give them an answer; you send them in [to hospital] without an answer. For continuity – you have already been through this already, and they do not have to tell you this story because you know this already. You know the name they gave their baby; what the room is like they had ready because you have been there with them through this.

PMA: How has this impacted on your relationship with the woman this time round?

MIDWIFE: It is a different starting point – multiparous women, because of their previous pregnancy have a different starting place. Continuity is important for everybody regardless of their experiences. At the same time, I am caring for two other women in similar situations. I have discharged one lady today with a healthy baby, but I did not look after them in their previous pregnancies. I had briefly met them, but I did not know them. The relationship is always different. You must be honest. I have learnt a lot about practice from these women and the most important thing is to acknowledge the baby that died as being part of their family and not ignoring them. There cannot be any awkwardness, you just have to ask. I got a thank you card from one woman that said 'thank you for saying his name', it's the most heartfelt and special card I've ever received. As for support for me, my team leader has been phenomenal. The day it happened [the still birth] the team leader was on a day off, but she just happened to be in the office. It was like she knew, she knew she needed to be there to scoop me up. It is also about looking for support from unexpected places. One of the parent ambassadors from the charity Beyond Bea, whose son, Henry, died contacted me on a separate matter and (with consent) I was able to offer his support to the father of this recent experience. It's important to acknowledge that I cannot fix things. I cannot make it better. I cannot alleviate anxiety. I can hopefully give the care in a way that suits them. Sometimes you do not feel like you are doing enough but it is enough.

PMA: Is there anything that you need to do now for you and your development? What comes next for you?

MIDWIFE: I think there is a fine line in most of midwifery – of being the midwife you want to be and protecting yourself. The two do not always go hand in hand. Giving yourself to the women does not always protect you. If I were not 'giving all of myself', I do not think I would be proud of the care I was giving. In terms of practice, we need to consider how we care for women who have had a still birth because we do not offer a case loading model of care. I go out of my way to offer continuity of carer and I probably end up going in my own time if I cannot fit a visit into my clinic time, because it is the care that they deserve. There is no continuity of carer team for these women. We have a bereavement team and continuity of carer teams, but they are not joined up.

PMA: What do you need to do about it?

MIDWIFE: I do not work in a continuity of carer team, and so if the woman were lifted out of my team, she would not have continuity of carer with me. She would have to explain her journey with her daughter all over again, when we already know each other. There needs to be a way to offer continuity of carer, but it is not as simple as setting up a continuity of carer team for women who have experienced a still birth because women may want to be cared for by their previous community midwife again.

NB: The restorative clinical supervision process does not provide the answers or solutions to experiences, but rather facilitates the person reflecting to find the answers within themselves in a supportive and confidential way. This reflects the Making Every Contact Count philosophy (NHS England, 2020) using open discovery questions.

## Service user feedback

Service user feedback is an integral part of UK midwifery courses and the NMC Standards state that 'a range of people including service users should contribute to student assessment' (NMC, 2018). Service user feedback is also used during the Revalidation process and should form the backbone of a professional portfolio and reflective practice to ensure that the service user voice is heard. The rationale for involving service users and carers is well supported and fits with the person-centred and empowerment agendas (Haycock-Stuart et al., 2016). The importance of acting on patient and carers' feedback was outlined in the Mid Staffordshire Inquiry, which exposed substandard care and a culture where patients were not listened to (Francis, 2013). The willingness of service users to provide this feedback is apparent. In a study by McMahon-Parkes et al. (2016, p. 205) participants felt it was valuable that the service user's voice is heard in the assessment of students. One participant said 'I was quite honoured to be asked ... sometimes as a patient you are not always included in everything'.

Practice-related feedback has been incorporated into the Midwifery Ongoing Record of Achievement (MORA), which has been adopted by many Higher Education Institutions in the UK and is a standardised document for student assessment (Midwifery Practice Assessment Collaboration, 2020). MORA aims to ensure there are clear goals for the midwifery profession as we transition into an autonomous and woman-centred relational continuity model. These goals are focused and aligned with person-centred models to ensure the sustainability of continuity of carer for the future.

The MORA document was developed with service users and asks:

How happy were you with the way the student midwife ...?

- cared for you?
- cared for your baby?
- listened to your needs?
- was sympathetic to the way you felt?
- talked to you?
- showed you respect?

These features align with the 6 Cs: care, compassion, competence, communication, courage, and commitment (Cummings et al., 2012).

In the context of the case-loading experience, there are some further considerations to highlight. Students and families will develop a much longer relationship over the course of the pregnancy, labour and the postnatal period compared to more ad hoc care episodes. Due to this relationship, service users may feel less inclined to give negative feedback and may overlook student's shortcomings. It is also a particularly vulnerable time in the life of women and their families, and some may be concerned about what will happen if they are critical of the care provided. it is also more difficult to ensure anonymity if the student had only a few women in their case load.

The recommendation to include service users in assessment was presented in the earlier 2010 NMC Standards and was subsequently reviewed (Haycock-Stuart et al., 2013). They found little guidance of how to implement this in practice and had reservations due to the power imbalance between practitioners and service users. Stacey et al. (2012) state that the term assessment infers a great deal of power and questioned whether feedback would be wholly genuine or would address the student's areas for development. They recommend that the terminology be badged as a 'review' rather than an assessment by the service user. It is also worth noting that service users will have had little preparation for this role and therefore the quality of comments may be variable. If feedback is not specific, students will be unaware of the areas to improve upon, and service users found it helpful to have both tick boxes and free text so they could expand on their answers (McMahon-Parkes et al., 2016).

Guidance from practice supervisors could help direct service users in giving specific and honest feedback as they could reassure families that constructive feedback will aid the students' development and will not have a detrimental effect on the care that they receive. They may also supervise this activity to ensure that feedback is sought at a time where parents will be most responsive and that this is done sensitively and without coercion, although the presence or guidance of the practice supervisor may appear coercive. It is vital that you maintain the confidentiality of service users in your documentation, therefore service users should be reminded not to write their names on documents or identify themselves.

The essence of service user feedback is summarised by Turnbull et al. (2013, p. 456)

> Service user involvement ... has the power to inspire students to take pride in addressing the little things that mean so much to patients. Practice-related feedback must be similarly valued by qualified midwives, not least because it may provide an insight into what service users value and aspects of care that need improving. Service user feedback, subsequent reflection on the feedback, and changes to practice, should ensure a maternity service that is truly woman-centred and responsive to women's wishes.

---

**Box 7.5 Activity 7.4**

Reflect upon the last piece of service user feedback you have received.

- How did you feel asking for the feedback?
- How did you get the feedback?
- What positive messages can you easily take from the feedback?
- What aspects show areas for you to enhance?
- How can you make a set of SMART(ER) objectives to take forward into your learning opportunities?

(Chapter 10)

---

**In summary**

From your deliberations to date, you may conclude that you need a range of experiences in a variety of practice settings to develop scope for future professional practice. Moreover, your experiences within your placements will vary depending on the model of care being used by the service and the women. Nevertheless, continuous exposure to practice is important to maintain a person-centred care approach from which to develop your practice from.

**References**

Anderson, T., & Davies, L. (2004). Putting the 'art' into the art and science of midwifery. *The Practising Midwife*, 6: 22–25.

Armstrong, G., Horton-Deutsch, S., & Sherwood, G. (2017). Reflection in clinical contexts: Learning, collaboration, and evaluation. In Horton-Deutsch, S. & Sherwood, G. (Eds.), *Reflective Practice. Transforming Education and Improving Outcomes*, 2nd ed. (pp. 214–238). Indianapolis: Sigma Theta Tau International.

Ashforth K. (2020). Exploring the woman-student-midwife relationship: A critical relationship on practice. *The Student Midwife*, 3(2). [online] Available at: www.all4maternity.com/exploring-the-woman-student-midwife-relationship-a-critical-reflection-on-practice/ [accessed: 13 September, 2020].

Ashforth, K., & Kitson-Reynolds, E. (2019). Fairy tale midwifery ten years on: Facilitating the transition to newly qualified midwife. *BJOM*, 27(12): 782–789.

Baird, B., Murray, R., Seale, B., Foot, C., & Perry, C. (2015). *Midwifery Regulation in the United Kingdom: Report Commissioned by the Nursing and Midwifery Council*. London: The Kings Fund. Available at: www.nmc.org.uk/globalassets/sitedocuments/councilpapersanddo cuments/council-2015/kings-fund-review.pdf/ [accessed: 28 December, 2020].

Bandura, A. (1995). *Self-efficacy in Changing Society*. Cambridge: Cambridge University Press.

Barrie, S. (2004), A research-based approach to generic graduate attributes policy. *Higher Education Research and Development*, 23(3): 261–275.

Bass, J., Fenwick, J., & Sidebotham, M. (2017). Development of a model of holistic reflection to facilitate transformative learning in student midwives. *Women and Birth*, 30(3): 227–235.

Berggren, A-C. (2003). *Hade jag inte last de dar artiklarna … Barnmorskors forhallningssatt till anvandning av forskningsresultat inom omvardnad* [If I hadn't read those articles… Midwives attitudes to the use of research results in caring]. Lunds Universitet: Pedagogic Institution.

Bolton, G. (2014). *Reflective Practice – Writing and Professional Development*. London: Sage.

Brodie, P. (2013). 'Midwifing the midwives': Addressing the empowerment, safety of, and respect for, the world's midwives. *Midwifery*, 29(10): 1075–1076.

Bryar, R., & Sinclair, M. (2011). *Theory for Midwifery Practice*, 2nd ed. Chippenham and Eastbourne: Palgrave Macmillan.

Butler, M.M., Fraser, M., & Murphy, R.J. (2008). What are the essential competencies required of a midwife at the point of registration? *Midwifery*, 24(3): 260–269. http://dx.doi.org/10.1016/j.midw.2006.10.010.

Byrom, S., & Downe, S. (2010). 'She sort of shines': midwives' accounts of 'good' midwifery and 'good' leadership. *Midwifery*, 26(1): 126–137.

Carter, A.G., Creedy, D.K., & Sidebotham, M. (2017). Critical thinking evaluation in reflective writing: Development and testing of carter assessment of critical thinking in midwifery. *Midwifery*, 54: 73–80.

Chief Nursing Officers of England, Northern Ireland, Scotland and Wales (2010). *Midwifery 2020: Delivering Expectations*. Available at: www.gov.uk/government/uploads/system/uploa ds/attachment_data/file/216029/dh_119470.pdf [accessed: 31 December, 2020].

Clarke, P., & Simms, M. (2012). Physical examination of the newborn: Service provision and future planning. *British Journal of Midwifery*, 20(8): 546–549.

Cook-Saher, A., & Wilson, C. (2020). Concluding reflections on building courage, confidence and capacity. In A. Cook-Saher & C. Wilson (Eds.), *Building Courage, Confidence and Capacity in Learning and Teaching Through Student Faculty Partnership*. London: Lexington Books.

Cummings, J., & Bennett, V. (2012). *Compassion in Practice: Nursing, Midwifery and Care Staff Our Vision and Strategy*. Leeds: Department of Health.

Cummins, A., Denney-Wilson, E., & Homer, C. (2015). The experiences of new graduate midwives working in midwifery continuity of care models in Australia. *Midwifery*, 31: 438–444.

Cummins, A.M., Catling, C., & Homer, S.E. (2017). Enabling new graduate midwives to work in midwifery continuity of care models: A conceptual model for implementation. *Women and Birth*. Available at: https://doi.org/10.1016/j.wombi.2017.11.007/ [accessed: 9 September, 2020].

Dalton, M., Keating, J., & Davidson, M. (2009). *Development of the Assessment of Physiotherapy Practice (APP): A Standardised and Valid Approach to Assessment of Clinical Competence in Physiotherapy*. Australian Learning and Teaching Council (ALTC) Final report.

Dawson, K. et al. (2015). Exploring midwifery students⬚ views and experiences of case load midwifery: A cross-sectional survey conducted in Victoria, Australia. Available at: www.mid wiferyjournal.com/article/S0266-6138(14)00244-7/abstract [accessed: 9 September, 2020].

Department of Health (2004). *The NHS Knowledge and Skills Framework (NHS KSF) and the Development Review Process*. Available at: http://webarchive.nationalarchives.gov.uk/20130107105354/www.dh.gov.uk/prod_consum_dh/groups/dh_digitalassets/@dh/@en/docume nts/digitalasset/dh_4090861.pdf [accessed: 9 September, 2020].

Department of Health (2010). *Preceptorship Framework for Newly Registered Nurses, Midwives and Allied Health Professionals*. Leeds: Crown Copyright.

Department of Health (2015). *The NHS Constitution: The NHS Belongs to Us All*. Leeds: Crown Copyright.

Department of Health, Public Health England, Royal College of Midwives, NHS England (n.d.). Midwifery public health contribution to compassion in practice through maximising wellbeing and improving health in women, babies and families. Available at: https://assets. publishing.service.gov.uk/government/uploads/system/uploads/attachment_data/file/208824/M idwifery_strategy_visual_B.pdf [accessed: 29 December, 2020].

Donaldson, J., & Gray, M. (2012). Systematic review of grading practice: is there evidence of grade inflation? *Nurse Education in Practice*, 12(2): 101–114. Available at: www.nurseeducationinpra ctice.com/article/S1471-5953(11)00156-9/abstract?code=ynepr-site/ [accessed: 9 September, 2020].

Donovan, P. (2008). Confidence in newly qualified midwives. *Br J Midwifery*, 16(8): 510–514.

Embo, M., Driessen, E., Valcke, M., & Van der Vleuten, C.P.M. (2015). Relationship between reflection ability and clinical performance: A cross-sectional and retrospective-longitudinal correlational cohort study in midwifery. *Midwifery*, 31(1): 90–94.

Fereday, J., & Oster, C. (2010). Managing a work–life balance: The experiences of midwives working in a group practice setting. *Midwifery*, 26: 311–318.

Fisher, M., Proctor-Childs, T., Callaghan, L., Stone, A., Snell, K., & Craig, L. (2011). Assessment of professional practice: Perceptions and principles. In C.E. Wergers (Ed.), *Nursing Students and their Concerns* (pp. 1–36). New York: Nova Science Publishers. Available: www. novapublishers.com/catalog/product_info.php?products_id=22965/ [accessed: 29 December, 2020].

Foster, J., & Ashwin, C. (2014). Newly qualified midwives' experiences of preceptorship: a qualitative study. *Midwifery Digest* 24(2): 151–157.

Francis, R. QC (2013). *Report of the Mid Staffordshire NHS Foundation Trust Public Inquiry – Executive Summary*. London: Crown Copyright.

Ghaye, T. (2007). *Building the Reflective Healthcare Organisation*. Wiley-Blackwell.

Gilkison, A., Giddings, L., & Smythe, L. (2015). Real life narratives enhance learning about the 'art and science' of midwifery practice. *Advances in Health Sciences Education*, 21(1): 19–32.

Gilmour, C., McIntyre, M., McLelland, G., Hall, H., & Miles, M. (2013). Exploring the impact of clinical placement models on undergraduate midwifery students. *Women and Birth*, 26: e21–e25.

Gray, J., Leap, N., Sheehy A., & Homer C. (2013). Students' perceptions of the follow-through experience in three year bachelor of midwifery programme in Australia. *Midwifery*, 29(4): 400–406.

Halldorsdottir, S., & Karlsdottir, S.I. (2011). The primacy of the good midwife in midwifery services: An evolving theory of professionalism in midwifery. *Scand J Caring Sci*, 25(4): 806–817. http://dx.doi.org/10.1111/j.1471-6712.2011.00886.x.

Haycock-Stuart, E., Donaghy, E., & Darbyshire, C. (2013). *Evaluation of Current Practices to Involve Service Users and Carers in Practice Assessment in 11 Higher Education Institutes (HEIs) in Scotland*. NHS Education, Scotland.

Haycock-Stuart, E., Donaghy, E., & Darbyshire, C. (2016). Involving users and carers in the assessment of preregistration nursing students' clinical nursing practice: A strategy for patient empowerment and quality improvement? *Journal of Clinical Nursing*, 25(13-14): 2052–2065.

Health Education England (2018). *Supporting Learners in Practice*. London: Health Education England.

Heaslip, V., & Scammell, J.M.E. (2012). Failing underperforming students: The role of grading in practice assessment. *Nurse Education in Practice*, 12(2): 95–100. Available at: www.nurseeduca tioninpractice.com/article/S1471-5953(11)00144-2/abstract/ [accessed: 30 November, 2020].

Hoffman, C., Dunn, D.M., & Njoroge, W.F.M. (2017). Impact of postpartum mental illness upon infant development. *Curr Psychiatry Rep*, 19(100). https://doi.org/10.1007/s11920-017-0857-8.

Hughes, A.J., & Fraser, D.M. (2011). 'Sink or swim': The experience of newly qualified midwives in England. *Midwifery*, 27: 382–386. http://dx.doi.1016/jmidw.2011.03.012.

Hunter, B. et al. (2018). Work, health and emotional lives of midwives in the United Kingdom: The UK WHELM study. Royal College of Midwives. Available at: www.rcm.org.uk/media/2924/work-health-and-emotional-lives-of-midwives-in-the-unitedkingdom-the-uk-whelm-study.pdf [accessed: 10 December, 2020].

International Confederation of Midwives (2017). *International Definition of a Midwife*. Geneva: International Confederation of Midwives. Available at: www.internationalmidwives.org/our-work/policy-and-practice/icm-definitions.html [accessed: 7 September, 2020].

International Confederation of Midwives. (2019). *Essential Competencies for Midwifery Practice, 2018 Update*. Available at: www.internationalmidwives.org/assets/files/general-files/2019/03/icm-competenciesen-screens.pdf/ [accessed: 7 September, 2020].

Joyce-McCoach, J., & Smith, K. (2016). A teaching model for health professionals learning reflective practice. *Procedia – Social and Behavioral Sciences*, 228, 265–271. Available at: http s://doi.org/10.1016/j.sbspro.2016.07.039/ [accessed: 7 September, 2020].

Kitson-Reynolds, E. (2020). *The University of Southampton Midwifery Values Based Enquiry Journey*. Southampton: University of Southampton.

Levett-Jones, T., & Lathlean, J. (2009). The Ascent to Competence conceptual framework: An outcome of a study of belongingness. *Journal of Clinical Nursing*, 18: 2870–2879.

MBRRACE-UK (2019). Saving Lives, Improving Mothers' Care. Lessons learned to inform maternity care from the UK and Ireland Confidential Enquiries into Maternal Deaths and Morbidity 2015–2017. Available at: www.npeu.ox.ac.uk/assets/downloads/mbrrace-uk/reports/MBRRACE-UK%20Maternal%20Report%202019%20-%20WEB%20VERSION.pdf [accessed: 20 December, 2020].

MBRRACE-UK (2020a). Perinatal mortality surveillance report. UK perinatal deaths for births from January to December 2018. Available at: www.npeu.ox.ac.uk/assets/downloads/mbrrace-uk/reports/perinatal-surveillance-report-2018/MBRRACE-UK_Perinatal_Surveillance_Report_201 8_-_final_v2.pdf [accessed: 20 December, 2020].

MBRRACE-UK (2020b). Saving Lives, Improving Mothers' Care. Rapid report: learning from SARS-CoV-2-related and associated maternal deaths in the UK. Available at: www.npeu.ox. ac.uk/assets/downloads/mbrrace-uk/reports/MBRRACE-UK_Maternal_Report_2020_v10_F INAL.pdf [accessed: 20 December, 2020].

McCourt, C., Stevens, T., Sandall, J., & Brodie, P. (2006). Working with women: Developing continuity of care in practice. In L.A. Page & R. McCandish (Eds.), *The New Midwifery: Science and Sensitivity in Practice*, 2nd ed. (pp. 146–166). Edinburgh: Churchill Livingstone.

McKibbon, K.A. (1998). Evidence-based practice. *Bull Med Libr Assoc Medline*, 86(3): 396–401.

McMahon-Parkes, K., Chapman, L., & James, J. (2016). The views of patients, mentors and adult field nursing students on patients' participation in student nurse assessment in practice. *Nurse Education in Practice*, 16(1): 202–208.

Midwifery Practice Assessment Collaboration (2020). *Midwifery Ongoing Record Achievement*. Health Education England.

Mitchell, J.M., & Davies, S. (2016). Implementation of a structured programme of preceptorship for newly qualified midwives in a maternity unit. *Nursing Management*, 23(6): 35–39. Available at: https://usir.salford.ac.uk/id/eprint/40947/1/PreceptorshipNM1463_R1.pdf [accessed: 28 December, 2020].

Muzik M., & Borovska S. (2010). Perinatal depression: Implications for child mental health. *Mental Health in Family Medicine*, 7(4): 239–247.

National Health Service England (2016). *Better Births: Improving Outcomes of maternity services in England. National Maternity Review*. Available at: www.england.nhs.uk/wp-content/up loads/2016/02/national-maternity-review-report.pdf [accessed: 14 March, 2020].

NHS England (2016). *National Maternity Review, Better Births: Improving Outcomes of Maternity Services in England: A Five Year Forward View for Maternity Care*. London: NHS

England. Available at: www.england.nhs.uk/wp-content/uploads/2016/02/nationalmaternity-r eview-report.pdf/ [accessed: 30 December, 2020].

NHS England (2017). *A-EQUIP Midwifery Supervision Model.* available at: www.england.nhs. uk/mat-transformation/implementing-better-births/a-equip/a-equip-midwifery-supervision-mo del/ [accessed: 28 December, 2020].

NHS England (2019). *NHS Long Term Plan: Online version of the NHS Long Term Plan.* London: NHS England. Available at: www.longtermplan.nhs.uk/online-version/ [accessed: 29 November, 2020].

NHS England (2020). *Making Every Contact Count.* Available at: http://makingeveryconta ctcount.co.uk/ [accessed: 9 September, 2020].

Norman, M., & Hyland, T. (2003). The role of confidence in lifelong learning. *Educ Stud,* 29(2-3): 261–272. Available at: http://dx.doi.org/10.1080/03055690303275.

Nuffield Trust (2017). *The NHS Workforce in Numbers – Facts on Staffing and Staff Shortages in England.* London: The Nuffield Trust.

Nursing and Midwifery Council (2006). *Preceptorship Guidelines.* London: NMC.

Nursing and Midwifery Council (2008). *Standards for Learning and Assessment in Practice* (SLAiP). London: Nursing and Midwifery Council.

Nursing and Midwifery Council (2009). *Standards for Pre-Registration Midwifery Education.* London: Nursing and Midwifery Council.

Nursing and Midwifery Council (2010). *The MiNT Project.* London: NMC. Available at: www.nmc.org.uk/globalassets/siteDocuments/Midwifery-Reports/MINT-report.pdf [accessed: 1 September, 2020].

Nursing and Midwifery Council (2015). *Revalidation: How to Revalidate with the NMC. Requirements for Renewing Your Registration.* London: NMC. Available at: http://revalida tion.nmc.org.uk/download-resources/guidance-and-information/ [accessed: 1 September, 2020].

Nursing and Midwifery Council (2015/2018). *The Code: Standards of Conduct, Performance and Ethics for Nurses and Midwives.* London: NMC.

Nursing and Midwifery Council (2018). *Part 2: Standards for Student Supervision and Assessment* London: NMC.

Nursing and Midwifery Council (2018a). *Realising Professionalism: Standards For Education And Training: Part 1: Standards Framework For Nursing And Midwifery Education.* London: NMC. Available at: www.nmc.org.uk/globalassets/sitedocuments/standards-of-proficiency/sta ndards-framework-for-nursing-and-midwifery-education/education-framework.pdf [accessed: 1 September, 2020].

Nursing and Midwifery Council (2018b). *Reshaping The Future Of Midwifery Education In The UK.* London: NMC. Available at: www.nmc.org.uk/standards/Midwifery/education/ [accessed: 1 September, 2020].

Nursing and Midwifery Council (2018c). *Part 3: Standards For Pre-Registration Nursing Pro- grammes.* London: NMC. Available at: www.nmc.org.uk/standards/standardsfor-nurses/sta ndards-for-pre-registration-Nursing-programmes/ [accessed: 1 September, 2020].

Nursing and Midwifery Council (2018d). *Future Nurse: Standards Of Proficiency For Registered Nurses.* London: NMC. Available at: www.nmc.org.uk/standards/standardsfor-nurses/standa rds-of-proficiency-for-registered-nurses/.

Nursing and Midwifery Council (2019). *Realising Professionalism: Standards For Education And Training.* London: NMC. Available at: www.nmc.org.uk/globalassets/sitedocuments/educa tion-standards/education-framework.pdf [accessed: 1 September, 2020].

Nursing and Midwifery Council (2019). *Standards for Pre-Registration Midwifery Programmes.* London: NMC.

Nursing and Midwifery Council (2019a). *Revalidation.* London: NMC. Available at: http://reva lidation.nmc.org.uk/ [accessed: 28 December, 2020].

Nursing and Midwifery Council (2020). *Principles of Preceptorship.* London: NMC.

Oxford Dictionaries Online (2016). Confidence. Available at: www.oxforddictionaries.com/defi nition/english/confidence/ [accessed: 1 September, 2020].

Payan-Carreira, R., Cruz, G., Papathanasiou, I.V., Fradelos, E., & Jiang, L. (2019). The effectiveness of critical thinking instructional strategies in health professions education: A systematic review. *Studies in Higher Education*, 44(5): 829–843.

Persson, E.K., Kvist, L.J., & Ekelin, M. (2015). Analysis of midwifery students' written reflections to evaluate progression in learning during clinical practice at birthing units. *Nurse Education in Practice*, 15(2): 134–140. https://doi.org/10.1016/j.nepr.2015.01.010/.

Pettit, A., & Stephen, R. (2015). *Supporting Health Visitors and Fostering Resilience Supporting Health Visitors and Fostering Resilience*. London: Institute of Health Visiting.

Phelan S (2010). Pregnancy: A 'teachable moment' for weight control and obesity prevention. *American Journal of Obstetrics and Gynaecology*, 202(2): 135.e1–135.e8.

PROMPT Maternity Foundation (2020). *Practical Obstetric Multi-Professional Training*. Available at: www.promptmaternity.org/ [accessed: 31 December, 2020].

Quality Assurance Agency (2012). *UK Quality Code for Higher Education Part B: Assuring and Enhancing Academic Quality, Chapter B3: Learning and Teaching*. Available at: www.qaa.ac. uk/Publications/InfoormationAndGuidance/Documents/Quality-Code-B3.pdf [accessed: 28 December, 2020].

Renfrew, M.J., McFadden, A., Bastos, M.H., Campbell, J., Channon, A.A., Cheung, N.F., et al. (2014). Midwifery and quality care: Findings from a new evidence-informed framework for maternal and newborn care. *Lancet Series on Midwifery*, 384(9948): 1129–1145.

Royal College of Midwives (2017). The gathering storm: England's midwifery workforce challenges. Available at: www.rcm.org.uk/media/2374/the-gathering-storm-england-s-midwifery-workforce-challenges.pdf [accessed: 19 February, 2019].

Royal College of Midwives (2018). The RCM standards for midwifery services in the UK. Available at: www.rcm.org.uk/sites/default/files/RCM%20Standards%20for%20Midwifery%20Services%20in%20the%20UK%20A4%2016pp%202016_12.pdf/ [accessed: 1 September, 2020].

Seldomridge, L., & Walsh, C. (2006). Evaluating student performance in undergraduate preceptorships. *Journal of Nursing Education*, 45(5): 169–176.

Stacey, G., Stickley, T., & Rush, B. (2012). Service user involvement in the assessment of student nurses: A note of caution. *Nurse Education Today*, 5(32): 482–484.

The Parliamentary and Health Service Ombudsman (2013). *Midwifery Supervision and Regulation*. London: The Stationery Office.

Thelin, I.L., Lundgren, I., & Hermansson, E. (2014). Midwives' lived experience of caring during childbirth: A phenomenological study. *Sex Reprod Health*, 5(3): 113–118. Available at: http://dx.doi.org/10.1016/j.srhc.2014.06.008 [accessed: 28 December, 2020].

Turnbull, P., & Weeley, F.M. (2013). Service user involvement: Inspiring student nurses to make a difference to patient care. *Nurse Education in Practice*, 13(5): 454–458.

Wain, A. (2017). Learning through reflection. *British Journal of Midwifery*, 25(10): 662–666.

Wallbank, S., & Woods, G.A. (2012). A healthier health visiting workforce: Findings from the restorative supervision programme. *Community Practice*, 85(11): 20–23.

WHO (2009). Global standards for the initial education of professional nurses and midwives. Geneva: WHO. Available at: www.who.int/hrh/Nursing_Midwifery/hrh_global_standards_ education.pdf/ [accessed: 10 September, 2020].

WHO (2019). *Strengthening Quality Midwifery Education for Universal Health Coverage 2030: Framework for Action?* Geneva: WHO.

# 8 Final project and quality monitoring

*Ellen Kitson-Reynolds and Kate Ashforth*

## Introduction

World Health Organisation (WHO) (WHO, 2019) pave the way for societal trends to influence advances in women's health care policy. As a student midwife it is pivotal that you develop critical and analytical competence so that you become a thinking user of research evidence to inform and enhance care provision throughout the childbirth continuum and positively impact upon health outcomes for women and their families. New and adapted maternity services need to maintain safe high-quality care provision to deliver that which it sets out to do (CQC, 2017) in a cost effective, resource savvy and sustainable way. It is therefore essential that midwives critically evaluate academic, clinical and professional performance using service evaluation, audit, quality improvement projects and research. As a result, midwives are required to utilise research skills to identify and propose solutions to problems to facilitate woman-centred care (NMC, 2015). This chapter will help students undertaking a final year project.

---

**Box 8.1 Activity 8.1**

Define and compare the differences between:

- Service evaluation
- Audit
- Quality improvement project
- Research

Consider how you could implement these approaches to evaluate/enhance your personal and local practice linked to continuity of carer/case loading.
(You may find Twycross & Shorten (2014) a helpful resource for this activity)

---

## Planning your final year project

You may be required to undertake a traditional dissertation or, more commonly now, an evidence-based project, systematic review of the evidence, service evaluation, audit, quality improvement project, a small primary research project or secondary data analysis research as a final year project. You will be spending a considerable amount

DOI: 10.4324/9781003051527-8

of time undertaking background literature searches, reflection on and in practice to justify your chosen topic and to contextualise it to identify gaps in the existing knowledge base. If you are embarking on such a project you will need to ensure that it is something that interests you and, more importantly, something that can be used to shape midwifery practice at both a personal and local level. It is unlikely that under-graduate research projects will be ground-breaking in terms of change on a larger scale, however this acquired knowledge can be used to support pre-work for future higher-level studies, a career in research, leadership and management, development and enhancing safe outcomes for all women and their families alongside your own continued professional development.

Examples of devising project protocols for both service evaluation and research are used to support understanding throughout this chapter. A fictious qualitative research (Corbin & Strauss, 2015; Mason, 2002) proposal for a pre-registration midwifery pro-gramme is considered, inviting you to contemplate the research looking at the views and experiences of student midwives working within one NHS Trust. The student midwives have had experience of working within both a continuity of carer model of care provision and a fragmented care system within a more traditional community midwifery team. Students are educated to the principles as set out through the Better Births (NHS England, 2016) and RCM (2018) national implementation agenda. Students appear to express surprise that midwives are not routinely providing continuity of carer models of care and have heard narratives from their practice supervisors and other midwives expressing numerous viewpoints on the Better Births agenda. Some comments concern anxiety linked to change, and students have acknowledged that with change comes uncertainty and apprehension for many (Corrigan, 2007). This led to asking how one cohort of students could excite their practice supervisors to embrace working in a continuity of carer model of care. The initial research aim was considered to elicit a positive continuity of carer experience for student midwives who would adopt this way of working in their first post as a qualified midwife. This research proposal was constructed to evidence the benefits and limitations of working in a continuity of carer team whilst being cognisant of the existing knowledge base on health outcomes for women and their families (Sandall et al., 2015). The students wanted the opportunity to compare health outcomes for actual cases to that of the literature to see if there was commonality in outcomes. At the outset, it is essential that the research has clear parameters to specifically address the final research aim and objectives. As a student project you need to be sure that the study is achievable in the time frame assigned to you.

Primarily a discussion was held as to whether a new service had been implemented already and if a service evaluation was more appropriate over a longer-term research project (Twycross & Shorten, 2014). If you find that you are unsure about which option to take, there are several things to consider as outlined in the Activity 8.2.

## Box 8.2 Activity 8.2

Now you have considered the differences between a service evaluation, audit, and research, how would you proceed with this project?

1   What is the question to be answered?
2   What are the aims and objectives of the project?

3   How will you undertake the project?

a   If you chose a research project, consider why and what this will tell you (see 'Choosing a research project' section)

b   If you chose a service evaluation, consider why and what this will tell you (see 'choosing a service evaluation project' section)

To help you decide, think about what the outcome/output is. What do you want to find out? Would you do one to inform the other hence, do both. What are the benefits of undertaking both to you and your sponsor?

Prior to starting any project, it is essential that you discuss your thinking with people you work with and people that are involved in the topic you are interested in. This may be charitable organisations, user groups, maternity liaison groups, colleagues, and managers at all levels. These discussions will shape your project to something measurable, achievable, affordable, appropriate, and useful to enhancing your practice, women's experiences and the maternity services at local level. It will also give you areas to consider that you may not have previously thought about or were unaware of. By reviewing the existing research evidence alongside, it is anticipated that you will critically reflect upon how this resonates with your experiences to-date of following a continuity of carer model of care and what this means for you in future employment as a clinical midwife.

## Background to your project

Understanding the current day practices may take you on a discovery of the historical policy and processes that have informed service design, delivery and inclusion of women and their families in modern day thinking. You need to consider seminal reports and research linked to your subject area. This is typically different to what you may have considered for your academic essays. You may have set yourself a set time range for literature searching, but you may miss key evidence that contextualises your project. As considered in Chapter 2, the Changing Childbirth report (Department of Health (DH), 1993) was pivotal in changing the philosophy of care to embrace a women-centred approach. This original five-year plan prompted a radical change to service provision which some 23 years later remains the topic of much debate. Better Births (NHS England, 2016) proposed similar principles to the original DH (1993) report but this time it appears to be enshrined in wider health policy with measurable goals. The emphasis remains on providing care for the woman throughout the antenatal, intrapartum, and postnatal periods through a team approach. This understanding of policy situates the topic area for further interrogation of the literature.

Formulating a preliminary question will guide your systematic search of the existing literature. Your library will have several resources and online training activities for you to access to support your learning and undertaking of a systematic literature search. Consider a framework to support your question development, such as PICO (Schardt et al., 2007), ECLIPSE and SPIDER (Cooke et al., 2012). There are numerous resources available to you to undertake literature searches and how to present your results such as PRISMA (2015).

Once you identify the best available evidence to answer your preliminary question you will be expected to critically appraise this evidence to identify what is currently known and highlight the gaps in the knowledge base, whist taking into consideration the quality of the evidence presented. Undertaking a review of the existing literature is key for both the service evaluation and the research project. So which approach did you choose in Activity 8.2? We are going to consider the final year project protocol now from the research perspective and then from a service evaluation viewpoint.

## Choosing a research project

The literature review evidence was also considered alongside what was known anecdotally from personal observations and acknowledging experiences in practice. For this study it was imperative to understand the views and experiences of midwives to propose how to make continuity of carer work for students to experience throughout their training programme. The research question was then refined as follows:

> How do student midwives experience continuity of carer models of care?

---

**Box 8.3 Activity 8.3**

- What methodology would you chose to answer this research question and why?
- Consider how you would gather your data to answer the question.
- Who would you want to recruit to answer your question?
- What do you want to find out from them?
- How will you analyse these data?
- How will you present what you have identified against the existing evidence base?
- What will you do with what you have identified?

---

## Methods

### Study design

Think through the differences between methodology, methods and design (NHS Health Research Authority, 2018). This research example followed a qualitative approach using semi-structured interviews with midwives and student midwives for data collection. An interpretivist philosophical approach informed the design and analysis as interpretivism lies within a relativist ontology in which multiple realities exist (Guba & Lincoln, 1994). Interacting with both midwives and student midwives during interview enabled the researcher to immerse themselves into the lived experiences of those who have experienced the subject area to apply an interpretation of individual experiences of continuity of carer (Ryan, 2018).

### Recruitment

Next consider how you are going to recruit your, in this case, participants. You may need to consider a purposive sampling strategy or a snowballing recruitment strategy to recruit participants. You will need to consider the potential for bias if you access participants in the same area that you are exposed to. Equally consider the benefits to interpretation if any. How will this be critiqued by your peer reviewers? Best practice will be to ascertain a 'gate-keeper' for the study who will be identified to protect potential participants from feeling pressurised into entering the study. Your gatekeeper will be the person to give out the related information so that you are not inadvertently, for example, accessing emails. Potential participants will be signposted to you as the researcher if they are interested in taking part in your study. This way their participation remains confidential to others.

Think through the inclusion and exclusion criteria for the appropriate group of participants to answer your question. You may have a screening information tool that may be used to ensure, for example, a mix of ages, roles and experiences. Participants will require a participant information sheet and be given the opportunity to ask questions and discuss the study with the researcher before giving their informed consent.

### Interview process

Think through where you are planning to conduct your data collection. Will this be in a university or NHS setting for example? For this research example, you may choose to undertake face-to-face, semi-structured interviews. You are encouraged to devise prompt questions or statements to support the interview process. You will need to consider how you will collect the data. This may be audio/digitally recorded for verbatim transcription or field notes recording. Consider what the benefits and consequences are for each option available to you.

### Data analysis

Depending on your methodology, carefully consider the most appropriate data analysis tool. For this example, an inductive thematic analysis using Braun & Clarke's (2006; 2014) 6-step framework is considered (Table 8.1). It is essential to consider how

*Table 8.1* Braun & Clarke's (2006) six-phase framework for a thematic analysis

| Step One | Becoming familiar with the data | Reading and re-reading of transcripts |
| --- | --- | --- |
| Step Two | Generating initial codes | Line by line coding of entire data set, developing initial codes |
| Step Three | Searching for themes | Codes examined for patterns and combined to form potential themes related to research aim |
| Step Four | Reviewing themes | Transcripts reviewed with themes across dataset to check accurate portrayal of the data |
| Step Five | Defining themes | Cross checking coding and adjustments to themes to reach consensus of themes and sub-themes |
| Step Six | Writing-up findings | Themes written up with specific examples from transcripts |

you are going to ensure trustworthiness (Guba & Lincoln, 1994) and you may want to plan discussions of emerging codes and themes with another researcher until the final themes are developed and agreed upon.

Consider if you are going to include member checking to ensure accuracy or to ask if the 'participants can see themselves in the themes identified' (Kitson-Reynolds, 2010). Reflexivity is an important consideration in qualitative research. As a student midwife with an interest in implementing continuity of carer models as part of your practice experience, it is important that you as the researcher acknowledge the potential for researcher bias that could influence the findings and to identify ways to minimise this potential.

### Ethical approvals

Research projects require ethical approval once all the details of your project proposal are finalised. Dependent upon the methodology and method of data collection will depend upon where you register for your ethical approval. Typically, this will be via your University or equivalent higher education institution and the Health Research Authority (HRA) if you are accessing patients and/or staff within a health setting (HRA, 2020). The HRA website has tools to assist your planning and to ascertain if you require both. Following this you then will need to consider Research and Development departments with the appropriate organisations and the requirements needed prior to commencing any project. These processes take time, and this will need to factor into any timeline for planning before any recruitment and data collection can be commenced. It is not uncommon for you to be required to make amendments to your proposal as part of the ethics process, and this will need to be factored in also.

### Funding

Typically, under-graduate final year projects are self-funded or conducted without any financial input. Research projects outside of this generally require funding through organisations such as the National Institute for Health Research (NIHR) (NIHR, 2020) or charities, for example. Any funding will need to be declared in order of transparency to reduce bias potential and possible coercion.

---

**Box 8.4 Activity 8.4**

It is often said that there is 'an elephant in the room' regarding the continuity of carer model of care and the links to stress and burnout. Reflect upon the key findings of this piece of research and

a   list the key areas that you consider beneficial/a strength to you as a practising midwife
b   identify what makes each of these a strength for you and your practice
c   list the key areas that would concern you as a practising midwife
d   using a strength based approach, devise a plan as to how you would alleviate potential limitations to your practice
e   compare your answers to b and d to identify a development plan using SMART [er]* objectives (NHSE, 2020) (Chapter 10)

*Specific, measurable, achievable, realistic, time bound, evaluate, readjust

### Choosing a service evaluation project

Following on from the literature review, you may decide to undertake a service evaluation. This example relates to a small-scale service evaluation required within the final year students' Trust where she undertook all her pre-registration midwifery education. Prior to identifying an area of practice in need of exploration the student had to understand the difference between a service evaluation and primary research. They used the NHS Health Research Authority's decision tree (2018) to determine whether the proposed project would be deemed research or not and, therefore, whether it would need full ethics approval prior to its inception. Fundamentally, participants were not randomised to different interventions, care did not deviate from standard care already provided, and the aim was to describe participants' experiences rather than make generalisable or transferable conclusions. As such, it was not considered to be a research project. University ethics was required to register the project. Processes were provided that differentiated the requirements for the service evaluation to what was required for research projects.

An initial reflection on practice and subsequent literature search found that an under explored area of practice was women's experiences of the latent phase of labour when they were planning to birth in a freestanding midwifery-led unit. This was to be the focus of the service evaluation (Ashforth & Naish, 2019). The literature search was key to identifying the research base of this area of practice and to determine whether there were any key concepts or practices not currently being adopted in a particular Trust. Identifying an area of practice and then honing that area down to a narrower focus via a literature search is pivotal when beginning the service evaluation as this search formed the foundation of the project.

A protocol was written as the modus operandi, setting out the evidence base, the aims of the project, and how the project was to be conducted step-by-step.

---

**Box 8.5  Peer advice 8.1**

A project conducted as a student will have to gain approval from both the Trust and the university, to check what is required from both and make sure you know who your point of contact is for both.

---

Your university will allocate a supervisor to oversee your project, so be clear about how much supervision will be provided, the role of the supervisor at each stage, and your timeline for each subsection of the work. A GANTT chart (Duke, 2020) may be used to assist in assigning deadlines, and other university and placement commitments could be added to juggle workloads and prioritise work accordingly (see Chapter 10). The method must be considered:

- how can you evaluate the area you are interested in?
- what are you hoping to find out?
- would a qualitative or quantitative method be more appropriate?
- If you are going to recruit participants, the recruitment process must be factored into the timescale as it can be time-consuming and may yield few participants (or none at all).

- If you do not manage to recruit any participants, how will you proceed with your project?
- Do you have time to conduct interviews, will questionnaires yield enough information for you to use?

---

**Box 8.6 Peer advice 8.2**

The service evaluation is a large piece of work, regardless of how big a sample or how many participants are used, and thus it should be an area of practice to keep you suitably interested over an extended period. Consider what you hope to gain from conducting the work: do you want to be able to use it to inform future changes to practice, do you want to use it in a future academic project (for example as part of further studies for a Masters or PhD)? While a service evaluation does not aim to evaluate experiences of changes to services, but rather to describe the service at present, the findings of the SE could be used to underpin a future change to practice or research project. Similarly, you will need to consider what your bias is. Prior to commencing the project, what are your thoughts on this area, do you have any pre-conceived ideas, are you expecting opinions to be one thing in particular? Any bias must be considered, acknowledged and mitigated against.

---

As continuity of carer is the main driving force for maternity services at present, it is an area that lends itself well to service evaluation. There are many areas that could be considered, with principles following either a quantitative, qualitative, or mixed methods approach. Table 8.2 sets out a few areas for consideration, along with method(s) of data collection.

The resources section provides an example of a contents page presenting the contents of the portfolio of work that was submitted as part the module assessment alongside the final written paper for publication to a midwifery-specific journal (Ashforth & Naish, 2019). The work was also disseminated to the local Trust so that the findings were used to inform further development of practice.

### Choosing a Quality Improvement project

Quality Improvement projects aim to introduce changes to practice that ultimately improve the quality of service provision. Such projects may be suggested, elaborated,

*Table 8.2* Considerations for future studies

| Area of practice | Method |
| --- | --- |
| Women's experiences of the current provision of antenatal, intrapartum, postnatal care givers | Qualitative – semi-structured interviews; questionnaires |
| Provision of continuity of carer: antenatal, intrapartum, postnatal, and birth outcomes | Quantitative – data collection from Trust documents and reports |
| The experiences of continuity of carer for a specific group of women, for example Brown and Black women, women with diabetes | Qualitative – semi-structured interviews; questionnaires |

and implemented by midwives in practice and may be a result of observing areas of practice that have room for improvement. *Better Births* (NHS England, 2016) is the driving force behind current endeavours to implement continuity of carer across UK maternity services. NHS Trusts must assess current services and identify ways in which continuity of carer can be expanded to meet national targets for women receiving maternity continuity of carer. Quality improvement projects focused on continuity of carer are a way for clinical midwives to bring about change that confers psychological and emotional benefits to women, in turn leading to physical benefits (Allan et al., 2018). Similarly, continuity of carer increases job satisfaction and reduces burnout amongst midwives (Newton et al., 2014) and hence such projects would aim to improve experiences and outcomes for both women and midwives alike.

An example of how a quality improvement project would do this, is by introducing continuity of carer to a pre-determined group of women. Three steps of implementing continuity of carer projects have been suggested as:

1    Audit current services.
2    Decide who will access the new continuity of carer provision.
3    Plan for implementation.

In this example, service provision in an NHS Trust has been considered.

## *1 Audit*

The NHS Trust is a large tertiary maternity unit with approximately 6,000 births per annum. Women can birth in one of four environments: at home, in a freestanding midwifery-led unit (FMU), in an alongside midwifery-led unit (AMU), in a labour ward. The NHS Trust covers an inner-city area served by community teams providing antenatal continuity of carer to women in community hubs, these women then receive their intrapartum and postnatal care from whichever midwife is on shift at the time. Continuity of carer is not guaranteed, and these midwives do not work on-call labour shifts to care for women in their team. However, if the woman's named midwife is on duty, they will be available to provide labour care for women within their team. In the same NHS Trust community area, women with social vulnerabilities are cared for by a team that specialises in extra support. These teams provide antenatal, intrapartum and postnatal continuity of carer across all birth environments. The NHS Trust provides care for women living outside of the city boundaries, with care given in one of five 'hubs' across the area. All women receive universal, rather than extra support, care parallel to that of women in the city without vulnerabilities. Each team has a specialist midwife who cares for women in the team with vulnerabilities but, unlike in the city extra support teams, these women do not receive intrapartum or postnatal continuity of carer.

An audit of current care provision for women in the five team outside of the city limits could make a reasoned case for a quality improvement project, ensure that a targeted approach is adopted, and act as a benchmark against which to measure progress. Areas for audit are suggested in Table 8.3.

The biggest difference between the city and non-city midwifery teams is that of care provision for women requiring extra support, as such this may be a useful place to consider a quality improvement project as it would increase equity of service provision for all extra support women across one Trust.

*Table 8.3* Suggested areas for audit

| Demographic details | Age, parity, language spoken, previous mode of birth if multiparous |
| --- | --- |
| Continuity of carer | How many midwives are seen antenatally, does the named midwife provide labour care, was the named midwife seen postnatally |
| Birth outcomes | Mode of birth, regional anaesthesia, place of birth, infant loss, stillbirth, IUGR |
| Women's voice | What do women think of the current care provision? |
| Midwife's voice | What do midwives think about the way they work at present, what do they think about care provision and continuity of carer where they work? |

## 2 Which women will access the new continuity of carer provision?

Continuity of carer has the biggest potential to improve outcomes for women with vulnerabilities or who belong to socially disadvantaged groups because they are most likely to suffer maternal and perinatal morbidity and mortality, although these are the women who are least likely to be offered continuity of carer. As such, and to increase parity of services across city and non-city teams, women needing extra support are the ideal group of women to be offered continuity of carer across the whole childbirth continuum. Women with vulnerabilities are more likely to disengage from care or access care late, both of which are associated with adverse outcomes, and by being able to forge a trusting woman-midwife relationship that enhances social and emotional support, maternal and perinatal outcomes should improve (Beake et al., 2013; Rayment-Jones et al., 2015).

## 3 Plan for implementation

The provision of continuity of carer can be challenging but rewarding (see Chapters 3 and 6) and so it is advocated that midwifery continuity of carer is provided by small teams of midwives. The non-city teams each has one extra support specialist midwife working within it and so an extra support network could be developed. This network would provide team continuity of carer across the five teams: each midwife would carry an antenatal case load, provide on-call cover for either two-night shifts or two long-days per week for all the women in the network's case load and be allocated flexible community time to provide postnatal care to their original case load and offer postnatal support to other women in the network as required. Continuity of carer rates would increase; birth outcomes and women's experiences of care would hopefully improve as a result. The midwives in the extra support network would be able to work flexibly to cover intrapartum shifts, they would have a support network of colleagues with whom they could share ideas, discuss concerns, debrief after particularly challenging experiences, and offer peer-to-peer supervision and support. Strong connections between members of the multidisciplinary team and continuity of carer are even more pivotal when child protection or safeguarding services are involved because of the need for effective information-sharing and collaborative working to ensure the safety of those concerned (Leap et al., 2010). Collaborative working across an extra support network coupled with continuity of carer should provide excellent clinical care and place the woman firmly at the centre of her care, which underpins the Code to which all UK midwives must adhere (NMC, 2015).

After the quality improvement project has been implemented and one cohort of women have experienced the whole childbirth journey via the extra support network, the initial audit could be repeated to assess the outcomes of care.

## In summary

Good luck in the planning and organisation of your final year project. Remember that it is better to plan and make a timeline/GANTT chart to help you to keep to your task. If you slip from your plan, make an appointment with your supervisor to adjust your strategy. Enjoy your project. You will learn a great deal from the experiences that will support you in your future role as a qualified midwife.

## References

Allan, H.T., Magnusson, C., Evans, K., Horton, K., Curtis, K., Ball, E., & Johnson, M. (2018). Putting knowledge to work in clinical practice: Understanding experiences of preceptorship as outcomes of interconnected domains of learning. *Journal of Clinical Nursing*, 27: 123–131.

Ashforth, K., & Naish, M. (2019). Latent phase of labour in a freestanding midwifery unit. *The Practising Midwife*, 22(8).

Beake, S., Acosta, L., Cooke, P., & McCourt, C. (2013). Caseload midwifery in a multi-ethnic community: The women's experiences. *Midwifery*, 29: 996–1002.

Braun, V., & Clarke, V. (2006). Using thematic analysis in psychology. *Qualitative Research in Psychology*, 3(2): 77–101.

Braun, V., & Clarke, V. (2014). *Successful Qualitative Research*, 1st ed. London: SAGE.

Care Quality Commission (2017). Driving improvement: Case studies from eight Trusts. Available at: www.cqc.org.uk/sites/default/files/20170614_drivingimprovement.pdf [accessed: 28 December, 2020].

Cooke, A., Smith, D., & Booth, A. (2012). Beyond PICO: The SPIDER tool for qualitative evidence synthesis. *Qualitative Health Research*, 22(10).

Corbin, J., & Strauss, A. (2015). *Basics of Qualitative Research*. Los Angeles: SAGE.

Corrigan, A. (2007). Continuity of carer and application of the Code: How student midwives can be agents of change. *British Journal of Midwifery*, 25(8).

Department of Health (1993). *Changing Childbirth: Report of the Expert Maternity Group Pt.1*. London: HMSO.

Duke, R. (2020). Welcome to Gantt.com: What is a Gantt chart ? Available at: www.gantt.com/ [accessed: 31 December, 2020].

Guba, E.G., & Lincoln, Y.S. (1994). Competing paradigms in qualitative research. In N.K. Denzin & Y.S. Lincoln (Eds.), *Handbook of Qualitative Research*, 1st ed. (pp. 105–117). London: Sage Publications.

Health Research Authority (2020). *Planning and Improving Research*. Available at: www.hra.nhs. uk/planning-and-improving-research/ [accessed: 31 December, 2020].

Kitson-Reynolds, E. (2010). *The Lived Experience of Newly Qualified Midwives*. Thesis. University of Southampton

Leap, N., Sandall, J., Buckland, S., et al. (2010). Journey to confidence: Women's experiences of pain in labour and relational continuity of care. *Journal of Midwifery & Women's Health*, 55(3): 234–242.

Mason, J. (2002). *Qualitative Researching*, 2nd ed. London: Sage.

National Health Service England (2016). *Better Births: Improving Outcomes of maternity services in England. National Maternity Review*. Available at: www.england.nhs.uk/wp-content/up loads/2016/02/national-maternity-review-report.pdf [accessed: 14 March, 2020].

Newton, M., McLachlan, H., Willis, K., & Forster, D. (2014). Comparing satisfaction and burnout between case load and standard care midwives: Findings from two cross-sectional surveys conducted in Victoria, Australia. *BMC Pregnancy and Childbirth*, 14(1).

NHS England (2020). *Making Every Contact Count*. Available at: http://makingeverycontactcount.co.uk/ [accessed: 9 September, 2020].

NHS Health Research Authority (2018). Research methodology. Available at: www.hra.nhs.uk/planning-and-improving-research/research-planning/research-methodology/ [accessed: 31 December, 2020].

NIHR (2020). www.nihr.ac.uk/researchers/funding-opportunities/.

Nursing and Midwifery Council (2015/2018). *The Code: Standards of Conduct, Performance and Ethics for Nurses and Midwives*. London: NMC.

PRISMA (2015). Welcome to the Preferred Reporting Items for Systematic Reviews and Meta-Analyses (PRISMA) website. Available at: http://prisma-statement.org/ [accessed: 31 December, 2020].

Rayment-Jones, H., Murrells, T., & Sandall, J. (2015). An investigation of the relationship between the case load model of midwifery for socially disadvantaged women and childbirth outcomes using routine data: A retrospective, observational study. *Midwifery*, 31(4): 409–417.

Royal College of Midwives (2018). *Position Statement: Midwifery Continuity of Carer* (MCOC). London: RCM.

Ryan, G.S. (2018). Introduction to positivism, interpretivism and critical theory. *Nurse Researcher*, 25(4): 14–20.

Sandall, J., Soltani, H., Gates, S., Shennan, A., & Devane, D. (2015). Midwife-led continuity models versus other models of care for childbearing women. *Cochrane Database of Systematic Reviews*.

Schardt, C., Adams, M.B., Owens, T., Keitz, S., Fontelo, P. (2007). Utilization of the PICO framework to improve searching pubmed for clinical questions. *BMC Medical Informatics and Decision Making*, 7(16).

Twycross, A., & Shoten, A. (2014). Service evaluation audit and research: What is the difference? *Evidence Based Nursing*, 17(3): 65–66.

WHO (2019). *Strengthening Quality Midwifery Education for Universal Health Coverage 2030: Framework for Action?* Geneva: WHO.

# 9 Transition from student to newly qualified midwife

*Ellen Kitson-Reynolds and Kate Ashforth*

## Introduction

Transition to 'becoming' a midwife (Kitson-Reynolds, 2010) starts before you apply to your training course provider. It starts at that moment that you decide you want to be a midwife; to be 'with woman' (Page, 2003). So why then is this chapter at the end of the book? Good question. Typically, many consider the point of registration to be the transition from one state to another (Jacob & Lavender, 2008; Kitson-Reynolds et al., 2014; Epstein, 2013; Eraut, 1994) however that point in time is possibly too late for people to 'hit the ground running' (Kitson-Reynolds, 2010) as part of an effective and efficient workforce. Even though transition to becoming a qualified midwife commences prior to the inception of pre-registration education and training, newly qualified midwives continue to experience a culture shock when they begin their first post (Kramer, 1974; Maben & Clark, 1996; Godinez et al., 1999; Gerrish, 2000; Montgomery el al., 2004; van der Putten, 2008; Kitson-Reynolds, 2010). The Department of Health (DH) (2010) and more recently the NMC (2020), advises that newly qualified midwives undertake a preceptorship period to ease this transition moving from novice practitioner (Benner, 1984) competent in providing universal care for women at low risk of complications to confident practitioners competent in delivering safe and effective midwifery care for women with additional care needs and within increasingly complex situations (NMC, 2019). Findings from a phenomenological study found that the real-world midwifery experienced by newly qualified midwives was misaligned with students' idealised fairy tale midwifery (Kitson-Reynolds, 2010; Kitson-Reynolds et al., 2014; Ashforth & Kitson-Reynolds, 2019). We all need to be better prepared to develop the confidence required as a new registrant and the realities of improving recruitment and retention within a positive culture and team (HEE, 2018; Lencioni, 2002). Incorporating a continuity of carer approach to your practice will support your transition to your first post as a qualified midwife and the future expectations of women focused care delivery.

---

**Box 9.1 Activity 9.1**

Before reading on, consider the following:

- Prior to starting your training, what did you expect your training to be like?
- What did your fairy tale of midwifery look like?
- How does it compare to your reality as a student?

---

DOI: 10.4324/9781003051527-9

- What problems do you think you will encounter as a newly qualified midwife?
- What do you think your life as a qualified midwife may be like compared to your life as a student midwife?
- Think about your hopes and expectations for the rest of your training, your first-year post registration and your five-year plan. What do you hope to achieve and where do you see yourself ultimately?
- Are their ways to keep your fairy tale alive now and when you qualify?

## Why is having a planned transition important?

It has been widely reported in a series of Royal College of Midwives publications that 'it is the responsibility of every NHS provider to ensure midwifery staffing levels are adequate to provide high quality maternity care' (RCM, 2018) however, the UK national midwife shortage continues. In England, the RCM highlights this deficit to be approximately 2500 whole time equivalent midwives (RCM, 2019). With the inception of Better Births (Cumberledge, 2016; NHS England, 2016) the then health secretary Jeremy Hunt pledged to increase student midwife numbers to address the shortfall in midwives to births ratio. This has not been without its challenges with the NHS, Health Education England (HEE), NMC, Council of Deans working together to increase the training numbers by 25–50% from September 2020, depending which part of the country the provider is recruiting to, whilst within a global pandemic (Willan et al., 2020) where NHS health care student placements have been slashed due to changes within, for example, maternity services and staffing levels have reduced due to redeployment, shielding or other reasons. It is widely anticipated to have a catastrophic impact on future workforce if students are unable to be supervised and/or even undertake their clinical practice placements, coupled with the fact that a significant number of newly qualified midwives leave the profession within five years of registering (Hunter et al., 2019; RCM, 2018; Hunter & Warren, 2014). There is a great deal of investment into the retention of the NHS workforce through the REPAIR project – Reducing Pre-registration Attrition and Improving Retention (HEE, Lovegrove, 2018). This report considers the need to develop the transition process to be supportive and nurturing with a closer consideration of the rollercoaster of experiences and confidence levels during the first year since registration (Kitson-Reynolds, 2010; Kitson-Reynolds et al., 2014; Halpin, 2015; Kitson-Reynolds & Trenerry, 2015; Kitson-Reynolds & Trenerry, 2019; Ashforth & Kitson-Reynolds, 2019). The Kings Fund consider having the courage of compassion when supporting newly qualified nurses and midwives stating that there are three core work needs: these being *'autonomy, belonging and contribution'* (West et al., 2020, p. 1). It is clearly acknowledged that the transition from student to qualified practitioner, if not sensitively considered, will contribute to attrition in the workforce. West et al.'s (2020) report outlines eight key recommendations for employers to achieve these three needs (Figure 9.1).

Transition shock is not a new concept, indeed, Kramer first recorded this in 1974. The NMC (2019) standards for pre-registration midwifery programmes addresses the concept of transition throughout each of the 'Domains' to be achieved. From a thorough review of these proficiencies, it is clear that much of what would typically occur in a preceptorship year will now occur in year three of a typical education programme and

- Authority
- empowerment and influence
- justice and fairness
- work conditions and working schedules
- teamworking
- culture and leadership
- workload
- management and supervision;
- and learning, education and development

*Figure 9.1* Eight key recommendations to address the core work needs (West et al., 2020)

preceptorship periods will need to be reconsidered to address the realities of the role. This is timely and has fit with implementation of the Continuity of Carer agenda (NHS England, 2016) as midwives caring for women and their families. As in Chapter 2, midwifery cultures are not always as conducive for the individualised care of the newly qualified midwife (Phillips et al., 2014). This is addressed through the new NMC (2020) principles for preceptorship publication. Reports such as Mind the Gap (HEE, 2015) have highlighted the current generations in the workforce in terms of 'generational differences'. Many individuals can see congruence with these linked to retention and satisfaction with their roles however there are a number who feel insulted by the nuances inferred linked to their generation traits. Despite this, many employers are utilising these generation traits to secure a longer term, high quality, safe workforce. Ensuring that you have a structured transition in a culture of compassion that is supportive in nature, will enable to you develop the skills and resilience for realistic, fast changing, often stressful but rewarding workload, to continue in the career that you have worked hard to achieve.

## Professionalism and professional behaviours

Professionalism considers the qualities connected with 'trained and skilled people to be confident, responsible reflective innovative and engaged' (O'Sullivan, 2011), and more specifically in a midwifery context as being 'characterised by the autonomous evidence-based decision-making by members of an occupation who share the same values and education. Professionalism in nursing and midwifery is realised through purposeful relationships and underpinned by environments that facilitate professional practice' (NMC, 2017, p. 3).

### Box 9.2 Activity 9.2

- Considering the above definitions, what does professionalism look like to you in a midwifery context?
- Do you think that it is easy to uphold standards of professionalism? Why/not? What barriers could there be to acting in a professional manner? What facilitates professionalism?
- Where do midwives' standards of professionalism come from?
- How do we measure professionalism?

Qualified midwives have a professional code of conduct to which they must adhere (NMC, 2015), which is essential to the provision of high-quality care and to the attainment of good outcomes (NMC, 2017). Professional behaviour is expected from the outset of midwifery training, and candidates would not have been offered a place on a training programme if they had been unable to uphold the standards of the profession. At the point of qualification and registration, midwives must embody the professional behaviours and practices as underpinned by the Code (NMC, 2015), upheld by revalidation, and recognised by their status on the Nursing and Midwifery Council register (NMC, 2017). These behaviours do not 'kick in' at the point of qualification, but rather training should be an ongoing process that enables students to become socialised into professional behaviours and practices in line with The Code. These behaviours should be role modelled to students by peers, practice supervisors, practice assessors, members of the multidisciplinary team, and their peers alike.

---

**Box 9.3 Activity 9.3**

- Consider your daily life, do you uphold your professional values and behaviours inside and outside of work? How do you manage this?
- Think about your use of social media. Do you use Facebook, Twitter, Instagram, and are people able to access these accounts? If women in your care saw these accounts, what would their impression of you be?
- Are these accounts professional in nature, for example do you use Twitter to connect to other students and midwives? Does what you say reflect your professional behaviours and standards?
- Do you think it is right that your personal use of social media should have to uphold professional standards? Why/not?
- Think of some things that may not be appropriate for you to post or discuss.

---

Each of the four pillars of the Code – prioritising people; practising effectively; preserving safety; promoting professionalism and trust – is pivotal in maintaining professional behaviours and optimising care (NMC, 2015). Three years post-qualification when it is time to revalidate, the evidence that you submit to the midwife or professional midwifery advocate who is witnessing and confirming your revalidation is based around the pillars of the Code and reflections must demonstrate a connection to the Code in order to prove that you are maintaining your professional standards. As such, it is beneficial to consider each pillar and its contribution to professionalism separately. Furthermore, it may be useful when reflecting as students to consider how aspects of your reflection demonstrate adherence to the Code in order that you become used to doing so.

## Prioritising people

Is the care you are witnessing and providing kind and compassionate, is it holistic and person-centred? The Code advocates that women are listened to and are included in decision-making about their ongoing care. Midwives are advocates for women, their right to access care and their right to decline care or interventions, which may be particularly challenging when decisions are being made that may lead to poor out-comes. Decision-making in midwifery practice is multifaceted, subjective, holistic, and may be influenced by practitioners' and women's experiences (Hastie & Dawes, 2010). For example, a clinician who has experienced a poor outcome in one situation may make more cautionary recommendations for care planning if they encounter a similar situation again to attempt to avoid another poor outcome. As such, cognitive bias may be introduced to the decision-making process. Similarly, women bring their own experiences, preferences and perceptions of risk to the decision-making process. This elevates the decision-making process from one that is unemotional and based on research-based evidence (Noseworthy et al., 2013). Decision-making in midwifery practice is based on partnership between the woman and the midwife (Ménage, 2016) and it is recognised that both contribute evidence to the process (Ashforth & Kitson-Reynolds, 2018). Furthermore, decision-making is not always confined to the woman-midwife dyad and may involve other members of the multidisciplinary team. This type of shared decision-making, situated firmly in woman-centred care, must be based on non-biased, evidence-based information, open and honest conversations about options, outcomes, benefits and risks (Coulter & Collins, 2011; Noseworthy et al., 2013; Ashforth & Kitson-Reynolds, 2019).

The Code (NMC, 2015) emphasises women's autonomy, which is underpinned by biomedical ethics (Beauchamp & Childress, 1994) and midwives may struggle when caring for women whose decisions or preferences threaten the status quo by contra-vening guidelines that may prioritise fetal well-being and maternal physical well-being, but not take into consideration women's choices or their emotional well-being (Symon, 2006; Thompson, 2013; Ashforth & Kitson-Reynolds, 2019).

---

**Box 9.4 Activity 9.4**

- Think of an example from practice when someone has declined care recom-mended to them by yourself, a midwife or a doctor, or when they have requested care that is outside of guidelines.
- How was that person communicated with? Were any tools used to aid her decision-making?
- Was the Code upheld, for example was the person's autonomy respected?
- What was the outcome, and could the situation have been improved at all?

---

## Practise effectively

Midwives are expected to practise in line with the best available evidence, work colla-boratively with members of the multidisciplinary team that includes obstetricians, health visitors, social workers, family nurse partnership, neonatologists, and keep accurate and legible documentation that is contemporaneous whenever possible. In order to practise effectively midwives must be able to communicate clearly, including with women who have additional communication needs. For example, women may have hearing loss or may not have English as their first language and require an interpreter.

**Box 9.5 Activity 9.5**

- Consider this example from practice and think about how you would have behaved in this situation, what could you or would you have done?
- Ana is a primiparous woman. She is at low risk of complications and is being seen by her midwife in a community antenatal clinic. Due to current Covid-19 lockdown restrictions, all women must attend appointments alone. The midwife has never met Ana before as she has recently taken over her care, although she has been told that she needs to arrange an interpreter for the appointment. Just before the appointment starts, she texts Ana to ask which language she needs to arrange an interpreter for. Ana's husband calls the midwife immediately and says that Ana does not need an interpreter as he will translate for her. What would you do at this point?
- The conversation continues and Ana's husband reports that he has been allowed into previous appointments as he is interpreting for her. How would you manage this situation?
- Ana enters the clinic, and the midwife asks Ana if she would like an interpreter, she declines. Ana's husband is already connected to Ana's phone and can hear the conversation. How would you conduct the appointment?
- What may concern you about this situation, and what might you do because of it?
- Consider how this situation could challenge your professionalism, who would you discuss this with?

## Preserving safety

In order to maintain safety, midwives and students alike must practise within their own limitations. Recognising your own scope of practice and asking for help when a task is beyond your competence is fundamental in providing safe care. Deviations from the normal must be recognised and timely referrals made, and it is important to recognise that while you may not know what you need to do in a particular situation, you know how to escalate concerns safely and appropriately. Importantly, midwives and students must be candid about any mistakes made, offer help in emergency situations, be able to competently and confidently administer drugs within your scope of practice, and safeguard adults and children alike by escalating concerns.

**Box 9.6 Activity 9.6**

- As a third-year student midwife, you are asked to see a woman with significant safeguarding concerns in a postnatal clinic at a freestanding birth centre.
- Why might you have concerns about this appointment?
- You are told that there are no midwives or support workers available to supervise the appointment, what do you do?
- Having raised concerns, you are told by the midwife in charge that you are the only person free to see this woman. How do you manage this situation?

## Promote professionalism and trust

In order to maintain professionalism, midwives are required to adhere to the standards set out in the Code. They are expected to act with honesty and integrity, have a sense of self-awareness that enables you to consider the impact that your behaviour may have on others, maintain clear professional boundaries, fulfil all registration (or university) requirements, and refrain from expressing personal views or beliefs inappropriately.

---

**Box 9.7 Activity 9.7**

- One of your practice supervisors that you work with arrives consistently late to clinic, does not adhere to the uniform policy, and smokes within view of the car park. She is a long-standing and well-respected member of the team.
- How do you approach this issue?
- Are you tempted to not escalate this? Why/not?
- What is the impact of this behaviour on you and others in the team?

---

## Coaching and leadership

Leadership starts with you. You are the leaders of your profession and the future of the modern health service wherever you practice within the international arena (WHO, 2019) where leadership is multi-faceted. Positive leadership cultures are key throughout all aspects of midwifery related practice to ensure high quality and safe performances at all levels (NHS, 2019). Reports by Francis (2013), Kirkup (2015) and Ockenden (2020) highlight areas of substantial poor practices, patient outcomes and public confidences which are analogous to a deficiency of strong proactive leadership. By considering your self-awareness (Rungapadiachy, 2008; Rose, 2012) and professional behaviours, you will be able to work alongside others to enhance quality service delivery and subsequently health outcomes of women and their newborns (HEE, 2018; NMC, 2019). There is a compulsion to comprehend how management affiliates in order to fully appreciate and accommodate leadership effectiveness within your own practice. A healthy respect for both management and leadership whilst understanding the systems, technology and resources within your professional role as a midwife, will 'strengthen your capabilities' (NMC, 2019). Achieving this will empower women and their families throughout the childbirth continuum.

## What is coaching?

Effective coaching builds resilient practitioners with great leadership abilities (McAllister & McKinnon, 2009). Throughout your time as a student midwife and within your qualified practice, you will be expected to consistently model professional behaviours by acting as a role model to your peers, junior members of staff and the multi-professional team, the profession, the organisation you are affiliated to and to the general public that you encounter. Coaching is a process of enhancing the performance and capability of an individual by focussing on the here and now rather than the past or future to achieve a specific personal or professional goal by providing training and

*Table 9.1* The roles of practitioners within a clinical coaching model (Bown, 2019)

**You as the learner**
  Take ownership and responsibility of your learning
  Lead and deliver care to a group of women and newborn infants
  Peer support and supervision
  Complete learning log to provide evidence for Assessor in practice
  Identify a learning need and facilitate a 'learning hour' to encourage reflective practice

**Coach (Practice Supervisor)**
  Any Registered professional can supervise you in practice
  Coach you by questioning rather than telling
  Gives feedback to Assessor in Practice on learner progression
  Takes overall accountability for the group of patients

**Assessor**
  Is a Registered Professional who will be signing to state that you are achieving all practice
assessments

guidance (Skills You Need, 2020; RCN, 2020; RCM, 2020). Domain 5 of the NMC (2019) Standards for pre-registration midwifery programmes asserts that you as the learner need to take ownership and actively take part in your own learning. Coaching in a clinical practice area strengthens your capabilities, motivating you to take responsibility for your learning in a non-traditional environment. The coaching model, such as Faithfull-Byrne et al. (2017), aims to support you to higher levels of performance through access to a multitude of health care professionals in an array of formal and informal environments. As a learner, you will be encouraged to adopt strategies to facilitate you to identify solutions to practice based problems in a safe environment.

Dependent upon where your clinical placements take place, you may notice differences to how you have previously been taught and have learned. There are many models of coaching to support you in a more independent, self-directed, and facilitative way of learning (Clarke et al., 2018), rather than using a lecturing approach (Jokelainen et al., 2011). Your practice supervisor (coach) will step back and observe your performance to allow you to lead and provide supervised care. There will be times where a more direct approach is required however, this will not be the typical approach to your development whilst using this model (Table 9.1).

Coaching skills (Table 9.2), incorporate a strength based approach (Saleebey, 2013), to target high performance and improvement in clinical practice by focusing on your specific skills and goals that you have identified with your practice assessor and may include:

- Questioning (Figure 9.2)
- Listening
- Reframing
- facilitation

## What is Collaborative Learning in Practice (CLiP)?

Collaborative Learning in Practice (CLiP) is a placement model, underpinned by coaching where learners are encouraged to take the lead in their practice, caring for their own patient group and supporting their learning through individually identified

How will I/you decide who needs care first...?

Show me how I/you do this...?

How can I/you do this...?

What skills to do I/you need to achieve this/ meet patient's needs...

Where/who can I/you gain knowledge/ learning from...

What support/help do I/you need to do this...?

How will I/you prioritise care...?

Who do I/you need to tell?

How can I/you ......

Show me how I/you record this?

Tell me....

Show me....

What am/are I/you going to do next?

Why have I/you decided to....

Is there another way/approach to do this?

What would I/you do differently next time?

What have I/you learnt from this?

*Figure 9.2* Suggested coaching questions (Bown, 2019)

daily learning outcomes. Whilst this is the gold standard some clinical areas set weekly objectives due to the acuity within the clinical setting and level of student need. CLiP is considered to have originated from Holland (Williamson et al., 2020).

The philosophy and principles of CLiP follow (Williamson et al., 2020):

- The art of questioning learners, rather than telling
- Use of coaching styles to suit different situations and levels of experience
- The premise that learners take responsibility for all the care of their patients
- Learners will access learning opportunities that support their understanding of their patient's journey
- Learners gain knowledge and competence by 'doing' as opposed to observing
- Learners step forward and qualified staff encourage the step forward

The aim of the CLiP model is to develop a culture of positive learning with compassion and kindness by:

- Developing learner competence, knowledge and confidence
- Enhancing the overall practice learning environment
- Sharing supervision of learners
- Improving the learner/employer experience with the aim of improving the quality and safety of patient care

*Table 9.2* Activity 9.7

| *This activity should be undertaken throughout your programme of education* | |
|---|---|
| Year 1 participation | • How can I begin to understand coaching models and how they will support me in practice and theory? |
| | • What are my responsibilities as a learner? |
| | • How can I begin to evaluate models to support my development such as the GROW model (Whitmore, 1992)? |
| | • What is reflective practice and how to embrace this? |
| | • What is my participation within the CLiP model? |
| Year 2 contribution | • What is student-led and peer learning? |
| | • How can I set and achieve learning outcomes of specific clinical opportunities, management and leadership? |
| | • How can restorative clinical supervision support my learning? (Professional Midwifery Advocate engagement.) |
| | • How can I support and facilitate learning for other more junior students/ learners? |
| | • Have I started to action plan and considered the development of skills to identify gaps in knowledge and practice? |
| Year 3/4 Demonstrates proficiency | • Am I supporting and facilitating learning for other more junior students/learners? |
| | • How have I linked my practice supervisor training session to my continued personal development? |
| | • How am I preparing for my first post and preceptorship? |
| | • What am I developing for my continuous professional practice and action plan for first post? |

From day one of your education programme, you are transitioning to be a registered midwife on the NMC professional register developing your own resilience for a future in a complex, challenging and unpredictable workplace (NMC, 2019; Hoverd, 2014). You are also part of the multi professional team (NMC, 2018b) being supported to succeed and address areas in need of attention when necessary. Feedback from a practice area illustrates the positive benefit of employing a CLiP model of learning to you as the learner and your coach in clinical practice such as you have better learning experience, linking theory and practice, opportunity to practise management and leadership behaviours and personal and professional development. The SSSA (NMC, 2018a) standards clearly articulate the ability of any registered health professional to support your learning in the practice setting. The coaching model empowers you to become a confident and proficient practitioner; to receive a '360-degree' (Fleenor et al., 2020) assessment from your team approach to supervising and assessing you in practice; giving you the opportunity to learn from several members of the interprofessional team, instead of just one and encouraging peer support and peer learning. Table 9.3 provides you with some areas for consideration across the duration of your education programme and beyond into your first post and is based upon one AEI curriculum.

## Professional development

Learning does not stop once you receive your registration and first post. Consolidating your training typically takes a year for most individuals within a supportive

*Table 9.3* Areas to focus my learning on linked to the year of my education programme (Kitson-Reynolds, 2020)

| Academic year | Content |
| --- | --- |
| Year 1<br>　Participation<br>　(MORA)<br>　Focus on Self<br>　(HEE, 2018) | • Have I read the NHS long term plan (2019) leadership and talent management?<br>• Have I read my professional code and related regulatory body standards?<br>• What is leadership and how is this linked to role modelling professional behaviours?<br>• What leader do I aspire to be like and why?<br>• Using reflection, what kind of leader am I and how can my style drive positive change?<br>• What is emotional intelligence and how does this influence me as a leader?<br>• How do leadership and management complement each other?<br>• What is a culture of compassion, kindness, inclusivity?<br>• What is 'team' and what is my role within it?<br>• What is the difference between Management and Leadership? |
| Year 2<br>　Contribution<br>　(MORA)<br>　Working with<br>　others (HEE, 2018) | • How am I developing my knowledge of improvement skills and how would I apply this to all levels of leadership in the NHS?<br>• How am I using evidence to further enhance my leadership personally, with women and their families and within a team?<br>• What is 'team' and how do I build (multi-)professional relationships?<br>• How does a budget impact upon quality care – comparing management and leadership?<br>• How does using political awareness and appraising policy to lead vision and its implementation?<br>• How do I communicate and negotiate effectively across maternity services and health and social care agencies to achieve a shared vision and/or quality care?<br>• How am I building my personal leadership and resilience in a day to day setting?<br>• Do I espouse a culture of compassion, kindness, inclusivity when working with others?<br>• How do I cope when having difficult conversations? |
| Year 3/4<br>　Demonstrates pro-<br>　ficiency (MORA)<br>　Improving health<br>　care (HEE, 2019) | • How do I lead a team/others?<br>• How is leadership in the organisation showing positive change?<br>• Am I developing management skills?<br>• How am I understanding, analysing and mitigating risk?<br>• How is my critical thinking developing?<br>• How do I review and enhance quality and safe care?<br>• How am I leading and learning from clinical incidences to develop self, team and organisation?<br>• Am I planning and delivering improvement projects?<br>• How am I developing my decision-making skills?<br>• How do I ensure a culture of compassion, kindness, inclusivity at service design and delivery levels? |

environment (West et al., 2020). You will be able to set your own individual learning objectives with your PMA and line manager (as appropriate). So how do we develop? On a day-to-day basis this typically is through reflection, however many practitioners appear to reflect when things go wrong. Most of the time there are no errors or near misses and therefore the challenge is reflecting on what and why this went well so that we can do more of the positive things in practice (Ashforth, 2020; Wain, 2017a; Bass et al., 2017; Embo et al., 2015). We don't go out to intentionally to do harm; we go to do good things so think this way and celebrate the wins. What did you do today to make you feel proud? (Small, 2000; Brown, 2015).

There is a body of evidence that considers practitioners to reflect two different schools of thought: good outcome but poor process and poor outcome but good process (Symon, 2006). As a health care professional, poor outcomes are not acceptable in a risk averse setting (Symon, 2006). As a newly qualified midwife it is beneficial to consider the reflection from a holistic perspective to identify what you could do better and what you have done well. It takes longer and you may feel tired when you transition to your new role and you need to set aside time to achieve these lifelong learning reflective learning opportunities.

As a student you will role model the practise of autonomous, professional, responsible and safe midwifery care that underpins the delivery of intelligent high quality compassionate, kind, women-centred, evidence-based midwifery practice. Embracing technological changes having vision and digital literacy to innovate improving health outcomes will support your move to becoming knowledgeable and skilled professionals who are competent and confident in practice. As a student start to consider what your first post will look like and start to craft your career. Plan a 1-, 3- and 5-year plan and consider how realistic it is and what the barriers and facilitators are to you achieving. Factor in your current life events and consider how you develop resilience in all that you undertake. Factor in your relaxation time and consider where you derive your emotional support for those days that feel more of a struggle.

---

**Box 9.8 Activity 9.8**

Ask your practice supervisors:

- What they wished they knew as a student that they know now
- If their training prepared them fully for the role and if not, should it have
- Compare these responses to what your expectations are and review if they remain appropriate

---

Once you have registered as a midwife you are required to keep a record of your development to support your revalidation (NMC, 2017) three years post registration (Fairley-Murdoch & Ingram, 2017). As a student you are developing these skills through your practice portfolios for the SSSA requirements (NMC, 2018a). Start to collate evidence of your professional development from the first day of your programme. You are encouraged to demonstrate an inquiring mind through reflection and lifelong learning; be self-aware; develop the knowledge and skills to ensure you are competent and confident in practice; through a strength-based approach possess self-belief and have self-efficacy. Include service user feedback to support this lifelong, quality enhancing development and your contribution to making services and midwifery practice safer for all (Kirkup, 2015; Offender Health Collaborative, 2015; Arnstein, 1969).

---

**Box 9.9 Vignette 9.1: What did I wish I knew as a student that I know now**

As mentioned, transition begins from the moment you decide you're going to be a midwife. Transition is about becoming, and becoming a midwife is not only about gaining a qualification and a professional registration. It is about acquiring clinical skills, finding out who you are and what you value, making friends and building a team, networking and sourcing contacts, honing your decision-making and clinical reasoning. I wish that during my first few months of training someone had shown me a snapshot of my life now. I wish I'd known then that I had the head, heart and courage right there. I wish I had known I would make the most incredible work family, that they'd always be there to pick me up and dust me down. I wish I'd known how much midwifery would make me laugh and cry and how much passion it would instil in me. I wish I'd known to trust all the incredible people who tried to help me, right from the word go. I wish I'd realised I was enough just as I was. I wish I'd realised how strong I was, how courageous, how determined, how passionate. That journey, that transition from non-midwife to midwife happens slowly at first, but in truth you become a midwife in heart and spirit far earlier than you do officially. By the time I'd qualified I knew I would keep moving forward, I knew being a midwife would be incredibly challenging and that the hours would be long and anti-social. I expected it; I was prepared as a student. I urge you to grab hold of every opportunity available to you and if the opportunity is not there already then make one. Join twitter and network, make connections that may enrich your career, broaden your knowledge and even open doors for you. Reflect. write. Reflect some more. Write articles and submit them to journals for publication. Go to study days and conferences, submit abstracts to speak at them, organise your own. Join the university's midwifery society, create your own if there is not one already. Travel far and wide, near and far, or stay at home but open your eyes and be receptive. Listen to what women are saying to you, feel the words they haven't spoken. Drink tea with friends, the ones who are your shoulder to cry on, the ones you spend an entire summer sat on your sofa with trudging through essays and dissertations. Refine your skills, reflect, learn, practise, then look forward to what's next. How can you refine your practice? What course can you attend? What interests you? What ignites that flame for midwifery? Never stop asking yourself 'am I the midwife I wanted to become?' if not how can you change and what help do you need. Take care of yourself, build your resilience, do not shoulder everyone else's problems all by yourself. Support each other, build each other up, do not trample each other. Remember to take a moment to appreciate how far you have come. The best piece of advice anyone ever gave me was this: treat your course like it is a three-year job interview.

---

## Preceptorship

The preceptorship or newly qualified midwife period is often fraught with challenges. Supernumery time and clinical relations are not protected and may be disrupted as ward acuity dictates, leading to increased stress (Clements et al., 2012; Foster & Ashwin, 2014). While length of time spent as supernumerary members of staff varies greatly, this is dependent on such demands within the Trust as acuity, staff levels skill mix rather than on the individual needs of the newly qualified midwife (Clements et al., 2012; Avis et al., 2013; Foster & Ashwin, 2014, Wain, 2017). Recommendations for practice are that newly qualified midwives are provided with an individualised preceptorship programme with choice of clinical areas of rotation, learning outcomes and supervising midwife or preceptor to oversee and offer support (Kensington et al., 2016). Individualised preceptorship may be difficult to facilitate but it should be considered whether your first post is going to provide you with the support and opportunities you need in order to progress from novice band 5 newly qualified midwife to more competent and confident band 6 midwife.

---

**Box 9.10  Activity 9.10**

- When thinking about your first post, think about your needs and your expectations of a preceptorship programme. What do you want to achieve, where do you want to work: obstetric led, midwifery led or continuity of carer teams?
- What does your Trust offer you: does it offer a preceptorship programme, how long will it last, what are you expected to do, what competencies will you need to have signed off, which clinical areas will you need to rotate through and how long will these rotations be, are there opportunities for progression, and how quickly are you expected to achieve band 6?
- Does your Trust have more than one hospital site, do you partner with a neighbouring Trust, are their opportunities across the Local Maternity Systems? Do you know anyone that works at the Trust you are considering, what is the workplace culture like, what sort of shifts/patterns are midwives expected to work, how many on call shifts are you expected to work, what support is offered to newly qualified midwife, would you be starting your preceptorship with other newly qualified midwife if in a small unit, is their opportunity for you to link with larger or neighbouring organisations?
- If you are in a continuity of carer team can you meet with other continuity of carer teams in your Local Maternity System.

---

It is important that the newly qualified midwife is supported in practice by a preceptor midwife who enables them to practice autonomously but who is available to offer support reflection and debriefing opportunities (Hughes & Fraser, 2011; Kensington et al., 2016). They are not the same as a practice supervisor when you are a student; you have the responsibility once registered; they are your guiding hand (NMC, 2018a). This newly qualified midwife-preceptor relationship is important for development across the preceptorship as the ability to connect with peers to share experiences and the work culture which must provide a friendly environment conducive to learning in order to capitalise on the preceptorship experience (Avis et al., 2013; Clements et al., 2012; Foster & Ashwin, 2014, Wain 2017) and invest in our future workforce.

### Box 9.11 Vignette 9.2

When thinking about where I wanted to work as a qualified midwife, the Trust in which I had trained was the natural choice. I loved training there and felt that the level of care provided meant I would be exposed to everything from homebirths to high dependency care and everything in between. The Trust is known to have a good reputation for its preceptorship programme although the specifics of the preceptorship change each year depending on service needs. My preceptorship saw me allocated to my own antenatal clinic in the community team in which I had trained. This enabled me to find my feet and then hone my skills whilst supported by a small team that I already felt part of. Alongside my clinic I spent my first six months in practice carrying out postnatal visits and providing labour care in both the AMU and FMU. During my second six months I continued to conduct my antenatal clinic and worked the rest of my shifts on labour ward 'obstetric led unit'. Due to staffing pressures and skill mix my short rotations through the high risk antenatal and postnatal wards did not happen although I have occasionally worked on these wards since. The order of my rotation was perfect for me; I consolidated my knowledge and became competent and confident in providing low risk labour care. After this I was then able to add more advanced skills to my repertoire by caring for women with more complex needs. The expectation was that we would achieve our band 6 at around 12 months post start of first post, which I did a few months after this. I found that there were lots of opportunities to practice and then have skills signed off, apart from suturing as I found there was often not enough staff to supervise me initially. That said, when I escalated my concerns to the practice education team, they tried their best to help me. I found the support throughout my preceptorship to be unwavering. Jaki who had been my community mentor became my team leader and my preceptor. She continued to be my safety net, but we did not ever work together clinically to begin with which I was sad about at the time. On reflection I think this was beneficial as it meant I could not fall back on our previous student-mentor relationship. The biggest thing that Jaki brought to my preceptorship was her never ending support and belief in me and her constant willingness to listen to me reflect and debrief. She is also the ultimate critical friend as I know that she will always raise points of concern with me and will always push me to achieve my full potential. The Trust itself has given me many opportunities to progress. Eighteen months after my preceptorship ended, I have been lucky enough to gain my NIPE qualification, complete my Newborn Life Support training work as a student link midwife for the community team and carry a case load of women in need of extra support alongside my universal case load. While some of my peers left the Trust to complete their preceptorship elsewhere others have completed the programme with me and then have moved on. I think there are pros and cons of staying and leaving and so I think everyone needs to think carefully about what they want from their everyday lives. Being a newly qualified midwife is challenging but having the right preceptorship programme and being well supported can ease the transition from student to qualified midwife (Figure 9.3).

### In summary

Now you have reached the end of this chapter and book, you may choose to restart again from the beginning as your knowledge, understanding and experiences will have

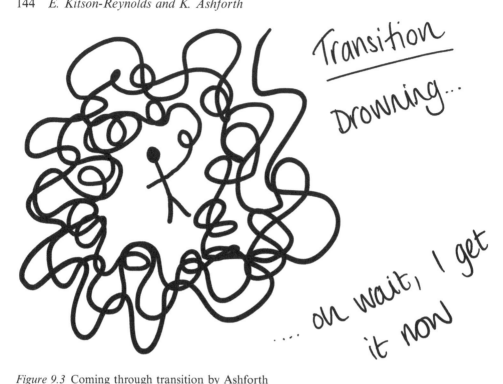

*Figure 9.3* Coming through transition by Ashforth

taken you to a new place for your learning and practice. You can also 'dip in and out' of the chapters to refresh your thinking and you can take this resource to your role as a newly qualified midwife and future as a practice supervisor. Good luck in the rest of your education and your role as a midwife providing continuity of carer for the women and their families you encounter. Enjoy!

## References

Armstrong, G., Horton-Deutsch, S., & Sherwood, G. (2017). Reflection in clinical contexts: Learning, collaboration, and evaluation. In S. Horton-Deutsch & G. Sherwood (Eds.), *Reflective Practice. Transforming Education and Improving Outcomes* 2nd ed. (pp. 214–238). Indianapolis: Sigma Theta Tau International.

Arnstein, S.R. (1969). A ladder of citizen participation. *JAIP* 35(4): 216–224.

Ashforth K. (2020). Exploring the woman-student-midwife relationship: A critical relationship on practice. *The Student Midwife* 3(2). Available at: www.all4maternity.com/exploring-the-woman-student-midwife-relationship-a-critical-reflection-on-practice/ [accessed: 13 September, 2020].

Ashforth K., & Kitson-Reynolds E. (2018). Decision-making: Do existing models reflect the complex and multifaceted nature of woman-centred contemporary midwifery practice? Part 1. *The Practising Midwife*, 21(10): 10–13.

Ashforth K., & Kitson-Reynolds E. (2019). Decision-making: Do existing models reflect the complex and multifaceted nature of woman-centred contemporary midwifery practice? Part 2. *The Practising Midwife*, 22(1): 9–13.

Avis, M., Mallik M., & Fraser D.M. (2013). 'Practising under your own Pin' – A description of transition experiences of newly qualified midwives. *J Nurs Manag*, 21(8): 1061–1071. doi:10.1111/j.1365-2834.2012.01455.x.

Bass, J., Fenwick, J., & Sidebotham, M. (2017). Development of a model of holistic reflection to facilitate transformative learning in student midwives. *Women and Birth*, 30(3): 227–235.

Beauchamp, T.L., & Childress, J.F. (1994). *Principles of Biomedical Ethics*. Oxford: Oxford University Press.

Benner, P. (1984). *From Novice to Expert: Excellence and Power in Clinical Nursing Practice*. Menlo Park, CA: Addison-Wesley.

Bown, N. (2019). Collaborative Learning in Practice (CLiP) Poster. Southampton, UHSFT.

Clarke, D., Williamson, G., & Kane, A. (2018). Could students' experiences of clinical place-ments be enhanced by implementing a Collaborative Learning in Practice (CliP) model? *Nurse Education Practice*, 33: A3–A5.

Clements, V., Fenwick, J., & Davis, D. (2012). Core elements of transition support programs: the experiences of newly qualified Australian midwives. *Sexual and Reproductive Healthcare*, 3(4): 155–162. https://doi.org/10.1016/j.srhc.2012.08.001.

Coulter, A., & Collins, A. (2011). *Making Shared Decision-Making a Reality: No Decision About Me, Without Me*. London: The King's Fund.

Cumberledge, J. (2016). *Better Births Improving Outcomes of Maternity Services in England. A Five Year Forward View for Maternity Care*. NHS England.

Department of Health. (2010). Preceptorship framework for newly registered nurses, midwives, and allied health professionals. Available at: www.networks.nhs.uk/nhs-networks/ahp-net works/documents/dh_114116.pdf [accessed: 29 June, 2019].

Embo, M., Driessen, E., Valcke, M., & Van der Vleuten, C.P.M. (2015). Relationship between reflection ability and clinical performance: A cross-sectional and retrospective-longitudinal correlational cohort study in midwifery. *Midwifery*, 31(1): 90–94.

Epstein, M. (2013). *The Trauma of Everyday Life*. London: Hay House UK Ltd.

Eraut, M. (1994). *Developing Professional Knowledge and Competence*. London: The Falmer Press.

Fairley-Murdoch, M., & Ingram, P. (2017). *Revalidation: A Journey For Nurses And Midwives*. Open University Press UK.

Faithfull-Byrne, A., Thompson, L., Schafer K.W., Elks, M., Jaspers, J., Welch, A., Williamson, M., Cross, W., & Moss, C. (2017). Clinical coaches in nursing and midwifery practice: Facil-itating point of care workplace learning and development. *Collegian*, 24(4): 403–410. https://doi.org/10.1016/j.colegn.2016.06.001.

Fleenor, J., Taylor, S., Chappelow, C. (2020). *Leveraging the Impact of 360-Degree Feedback*, 2nd ed. Oakland: Berrett-Koehler Publishers, Inc.

Foster, J., & Ashwin, C. (2014). Newly qualified midwives' experiences of preceptorship: A qualitative study MIDIRS. *Midwifery Digest*, 24(2): 151–157.

Francis, R. QC (2013). *Report of the Mid Staffordshire NHS Foundation Trust Public Inquiry – Executive Summary*. London: Crown Copyright.

Gerrish, K. (2000). Still fumbling along? A comparative study of the newly qualified nurse's perception of the transition from student to qualified nurse. *J Adv Nurs*, 32(2): 473–480.

Godinez, G., Schweiger, J., Gruver, J., Ryan, P. (1999). Role transition from graduate to staff nurse: A qualitative analysis. *J Nurses Staff Dev*, 15(3): 97–110.

Halpin, Y. (2015). *Newly Qualified Nurse Transition: Stress Experiences and Stress-Mediating Factors – A Longitudinal Study*. A thesis submitted for Doctor of Philosophy, London South Bank University.

Hastie, R., & Dawes, R. (2010). *Rational Choice in an Uncertain World*. London: Sage Publications.

Health Education England (2015). Mind the gap: Exploring the needs of early career nurses and midwives in the workplace. London: Health Education England. Available at: www.nhsemp loyers.org/news/2015/08/mind-the-gap-exploring-the-needs-of-early-career-nurses-and-midwives [accessed: July 2018].

Health Education England (2018). *Maximising Leadership Learning In The Pre-Registration Health Care Curricula*. London: Health Education England.

Health Education England (2018). *Repair: Reducing Pre-Registration Attrition and Improving Retention.* London: Health Education England. Available at: www.hee.nhs.uk/our-work/redu cing-pre-registration-attrition-improving-retention [accessed: 30 November, 2020].

Hoverd, B. (2014). *Powering through Pressure: Building Resilience for when Work gets Tough.* Harlow: Pearson Education Ltd.

Hughes, A., & Fraser, D. (2011). 'There are guiding hands and there are controlling hands': Student midwives' experiences of mentorship in the UK. *Midwifery*, 27(6): 786–792.

Hughes, A.J., & Fraser, D.M. (2011). 'Sink or swim': The experience of newly qualified midwives in England. *Midwifery*, 27: 382–386. http://dx.doi.1016/jmidw.2011.03.012.

Hunter, B., Fenwick, J., Sidebotham, M., & Henley, J. (2019). Midwives in the United Kingdom: Levels of burnout, depression, anxiety and stress and associated predictors. *Midwifery*, 79: 102526.

Hunter, B., & Warren, L. (2014). Midwives' experiences of workplace resilience . *Midwifery*, 30: 926–934.

Jacob, S., & Lavender, T. (2008). *Preparing for Professional Practice.* London: Quay Books.

Jokelainen, M., Turunen, H., Tossavainen, K., Jamookeeah, D., & Coco, K. (2011). A systematic review of mentoring nursing students in clinical placements. *J Clin Nurs*, 2(19-20): 2854–2867. doi:10.1111/j.1365-2702.2010.03571.x.

Kensington, M., Campbell, N., Gray, E., Dixon, L., Tumilty, E., Pairman, S., Calvert, S., & Lennox, S. (2016). New Zealand's midwifery profession: Embracing graduate midwives' transition to practice. *New Zealand College of Midwives Journal*, 52 :20–25. https://doi.org/10. 12784/ nzcomjnl52.2016.3.20–25.

Kirkup, B. (2015). *The Report of the Morecambe Bay Investigation.* Preston: Morecambe Bay Investigation Copyright.

Kitson-Reynolds, E. (2020). *Bachelor of Science (HONS) Midwifery Coaching Skills Through the Curriculum. What is Coaching?* Southampton, University of Southampton.

Kitson-Reynolds, E. (2010). *The Lived Experience of Newly Qualified Midwives*, thesis, University of Southampton.

Kitson-Reynolds, E., & Trenerry, A. (2015). Transition to midwifery: Collaborative working between university and maternity services. *British Journal of Midwifery*, 23(7).

Kitson-Reynolds, E., & Trenerry, A. (2019). The United Kingdom. In M. Gray, E. Kitson-Reynolds & A. Cummings (Eds.), *Starting Life as a Midwife: An International Review of Transition from Student to Practitioner.* Springer.

Kitson-Reynolds, E, Cluett E., & le May A. (2014). Fairy tale midwifery – fact or fiction: The lived experiences of newly qualified midwives. *British Journal of Midwifery*, 22(9): 660–668. https://doi.org/10.12968/ bjom.2014.22.9.660.

Kramer, M. (1974). Reality shock: Why nurses leave nursing California. The CV Mosby Company.

Lencioni, P. (2002). *The Five Dysfunctions of a Team.* San Francisco: Jossey-Bass.

Maben, J., & Clark, J.M. (1996). Making the transition from student to staff nurse. *Nurs Times*, 92(44): 28–31.

McAllister, M., & McKinnon, J. (2009). The importance of teaching and learning resilience in the health disciplines: A critical review of the literature. *Nurse Education Today*, 29(4): 371–379.

Ménage, D. (2016). A model for evidence-based decision-making in midwifery care. Part 2. *British Journal of Midwifery*, 24(2): 137–143.

Montgomery, E., McCandlish, R., & Martin, A. (2004). What happens after graduation? The WHAG study. A longitudinal cohort study of pre-registration midwifery graduates. *MIDIRS Midwifery Digest*, 14(3): 422–424.

National Health Service England (2016). *Better Births: Improving Outcomes of Maternity Services in England. National Maternity Review.* Available at: www.england.nhs.uk/wp-content/up loads/2016/02/national-maternity-review-report.pdf [accessed: 14 March, 2020].

NHS England (2019). *NHS Long Term Plan: Online version of the NHS Long Term Plan.* London: NHS England [online] Available at: www.longtermplan.nhs.uk/online-version/ [accessed: 29 November, 2020].

Noseworthy, A., Phibbs, S., & Benn, C. (2013). Towards a relational model of decision-making in midwifery care. *Midwifery*, 29: e42–e48.

Nursing and Midwifery Council (2015/2018). *The Code: Standards of Conduct, Performance and Ethics for Nurses and Midwives.* London: NMC.

Nursing and Midwifery Council (2017). *Revalidation: How to REVALIDATE with the NMC. Requirements for Renewing your Registration.* London: NMC. Available at: http://revalidation. nmc.org.uk/download-resources/guidance-and-information/ [accessed: 1 September, 2020].

Nursing and Midwifery Council (2018a). *Part 2: Standards for Student Supervision and Assessment.* London: NMC.

Nursing and Midwifery Council (2018b). *Realising Professionalism: Standards for Education and Training: Part 1: Standards Framework for Nursing and Midwifery Education.* London: NMC. Available at: www.nmc.org.uk/globalassets/sitedocuments/standards-of-proficiency/standards-framework-for-nursing-and-midwifery-education/education-framework.pdf [accessed: 1 September, 2020].

Nursing and Midwifery Council (2019). *Standards for Pre-Registration Midwifery programmes.* London: NMC.

Nursing and Midwifery Council (2020). *Principles of Preceptorship.* London: NMC.

O'Sullivan, M. (2011). Develop the Cambridge learner attributes [online] Available at: www.cambridgeinternational.org/Images/417069-developing-the-cambridge-learner-attributes-.pdf [accessed: 31 December, 2020].

Ockenden, D. (2020). Ockenden Report. *Emerging Findings and Recommendations from the Independent Review of Maternity Services at the Shrewsbury and Telford Hospital NHS Trust.* London, HMSO.

Offender Health Collaborative (2015). *Liaison and Diversion Manager and Practitioner Resource: Service User Involvement.* Leeds: NHS England.

Page, L. (2003). One-to-one midwifery: Restoring the 'with woman' relationship in midwifery. *Journal of Midwifery & Women's Health*, 48(2): 119–125.

Phillips, C. et al (2014). A secondary data analysis examining the needs of graduate nurses in their transition to a new role. *Nurse Education in Practice*, 14: 106–111.

Rose, C. (Ed.) (2012). *Self-awareness and Personal Development Resources for Psychotherapists and Counsellors.* Basingstoke: Palgrave Macmillan.

Royal College of Midwives (2018). *State of Maternity Services Report 2018 – England.* Available at: www. rcm.org.uk/sites/default/files/ENGLAND%20SOMS%202018%20-%20FINAL%20%2803.09.2018%29.pdf [accessed: 19 February, 2019].

Royal College of Midwives (2019). England short of almost 2500 midwives, new birth figures confirm. Available at: www.rcm.org.uk/news-views/rcm-opinion/2019/england-short-of-almost-2-500-midwives-new-birth-figures-confirm/ [accessed: 19 September, 2020].

Royal College of Midwives (2020). Welcome to I Learn. Available at: www.ilearn.rcm.org.uk/ [accessed: 19 August, 2020].

Royal College of Nursing (2020). Using a coaching model in practice supervision. Available at: www.rcn.org.uk/professional-development/practice-based-learning/innovations-from-around-the-uk/using-a-coaching-model-in-practice-supervision [accessed: 19 August, 2020].

Rungapadiachy, D.M. (2008). *Self-awareness in Healthcare.* Basingstoke: Palgrave Macmillan.

Saleebey, D. (Ed.) (2013). *The Strengths Perspective in Social Work Practice*, 6th ed. Boston, MA: Allyn and Bacon.

Skills you need (2020). What is coaching? Available at: www.skillsyouneed.com/learn/coaching.html [accessed: 28 December, 2020].

Small, H. (2000). Proud. Lyrics available at: www.metrolyrics.com/proud-lyrics-heather-small.html [accessed: 31 December, 2020].

Symon, A. (2006). Risk and choice, knowledge and control. In Symon, A. (Ed.), *Risk and Choice in Maternity Care*. London: Churchill Livingstone Elsevier.

Thompson, A. (2013). Midwives' experiences of caring for women whose requests are not within clinical policies and guidelines. *British Journal of Midwifery*, 21(8): 564–570.

van der Putten, D. (2008). The lived experience of newly qualified midwives: A qualitative study. *British Journal of Midwifery*, 16(6): 348–358.

Wain, A. (2017). Examining the lived experiences of newly qualified midwives during their preceptorship. *British Journal of Midwifery*, 25(7): 451–457.

Wain, A. (2017a). Learning through reflection. *British Journal of Midwifery*, 25(10): 662–666.

West, M., Topakas, A., & Dawson, J. (2014). Climate and culture for health care performance. In *The Oxford Handbook of Organizational Climate and Culture* (pp. 335–359). Available at: https://doi.org/10.1093/oxfordhb/9780199860715.013.0018 [accessed: 28 December, 2020].

Whitmore, J. (1992). *Coaching for Performance: GROWing people, Performance and Purpose*. London: Nicholas Brearley.

WHO (2019). *Strengthening Quality Midwifery Education for Universal Health Coverage 2030: Framework for Action?* Geneva: WHO.

Willan, J., King, A.J., Jeffery, K., & Bienz, N. (2020). Challenges for NHS hospitals during Covid-19 epidemic. *The British Medical Journal*, 368: m1117. doi:10.1136/bmj.m1117.

Williamson, G.R., Plowright, H., Kanec, A., Bunced, J., Clarke, D., Jamisone, C. (2020). Collaborative learning in practice: A systematic review and narrative synthesis of the research evidence in nurse education. *Nurse Education In Practice*, 43: 102706.

# 10 Resources

*Ellen Kitson-Reynolds and Kate Ashforth*

Chapter 10 contains practical resources, such as work sheets and 'journeys' that have been referred to within previous chapters. These resources are available to you as a template that can be adapted to be meaningful to you and your own programme of midwifery education and are based upon examples from one university and from the evidence base. These are not meant to replace your AEI documentation, but complement or highlight nuances between different autonomous practicing midwives. They are and aide to supporting your development throughout your training and for you to consider as a practice supervisor when supporting future learners.

## Chapter 1

*Table 10.1a* Kitson-Reynolds (2020) VBE journey Year One

| Order of sessions | Cummings and Bennett 6Cs (2012) focus | Session theme | | Principles – During this session you will: |
|---|---|---|---|---|
| 1 | Communication, compassion, courage, care, commitment, competence | 1 | Welcome and getting to know each other | • Ground rules |
| | | | | • Meeting and greeting |
| | | | | • What I am feeling about this level of education? |
| | | 2 | Disorientation in learning | • Why should I participate? |
| | | | | • Being vulnerable/self-awareness |
| | | | | • Strengthen your capabilities |
| | | | | • Confusion and disorientation, overwhelming |
| | | | | • Change of self, true to self |
| 2 | Communication, compassion, courage, care, commitment, competence | 1 | What kind of midwife do I want to be? | • Getting to know and understand yourself |
| | | | | • Who are you, looking at values, your journey getting here? |
| | | 2 | What is professionalism? [in academic and practice settings] | • Timekeeping |
| | | | | • Behaviours |
| | | | | • Responsibility |
| | | | | • Mind the gap report |
| | | | | • Job versus being a student |
| | | | | • Personal leadership |
| | | | | • Strength based approach |
| | | | | • Dealing with my own distress |

DOI: 10.4324/9781003051527-10

| Order of sessions | Cummings and Bennett 6Cs (2012) focus | | Session theme | Principles – During this session you will: |
|---|---|---|---|---|
| 3 | Communication, compassion, courage, care, commitment, competence | 1 | Recognising the values of others | • Begin to understand how personal values impact on others |
| | | 2 | Introducing Multi professional working (IPE) | • Begin to recognise the values of others and how this may impact on behaviour |
| | | | | • Consider the interactions between professional and personal values in nursing and midwifery and the potential impact on client care |
| | | | | • Choose a profession that you would like to explore that you are likely to encounter as a midwife and produce a presentation for your group |
| | | | | • Developing coaching skills awareness |
| 4 | Courage | 1 | Challenging perceptions and behaviours: case study | • Interactions between professionals, peers and public |
| | | | | • Impact on outcomes of care |
| | | 2 | Feminism/ humanism | • Personalities |
| | | | | • Professional relationships |
| | | | | • Languaging |
| | | | | • Ageism |
| | | | | • Prejudice |
| | | | | • Status quo - challenging the norm |
| | | | | • Language used from mothers to children |
| | | | | • Midwifery culture/radical candour |
| | | | | • Feelings wheel |
| 5 | Communication | 1 | Videoed scenario | • Developing self-awareness |
| | | | | • Developing critical friend skills |
| | | | | • Seeing yourself as others see you |
| | | | | • Strengths and areas for enhancement |
| 6 | Compassion | 1 | How have I/ my values changed since my exposure to practice and | • Self-awareness |
| | | | | • Acceptance |
| | | | | • Myers Briggs |
| | | | | • Reflection on practice [Schon] |
| | | 2 | Developing resilience | • Lean in |
| 7 | Communication, compassion, courage, care, commitment, competence | 1 | MECC 1 | • Developing questioning skills |
| | | 2 | Difficult conversations/ asking difficult questions | • Developing listening skills |
| | | | | • Non-verbal cues |
| | | | | • Timing |
| | | | | • Empathy |
| | | | | • Environments |

| Order of sessions | Cummings and Bennett 6Cs (2012) focus | Session theme | Principles – During this session you will: |
|---|---|---|---|
| 8 | Courage | 1  MECC 2 | • Interactions between professionals, peers and public<br>• Impact on outcomes of care<br>• Developing questioning skills<br>• Developing listening skills<br>• Facilitating changing and challenging health perceptions |
| Practice experience 1 | Communication, compassion, courage, care, commitment, competence | Journal club 1 | • Reviewing evidence based practice<br>• Research into practice<br>• How to apply a critical appraisal to evidence<br>• Considering the gaps in knowledge<br>• Developing research understanding and language<br>• How to relate research to client care planning |
| Practice experience 2 | Communication, compassion, courage, care, commitment, competence | Journal club 2 | • Reviewing evidence based practice<br>• Research into practice<br>• How to apply a critical appraisal to evidence<br>• Considering the gaps in knowledge<br>• Developing research understanding and language<br>• How to relate research to client care planning |

*Table 10.1b* Integrating multi professional learning (MPL) in midwifery using the VBE process

| Recognising values of others - Introduce MPL integration – set up for presentations in week | Difficult conversations – What is professionalism and how does it impact on your practice |
|---|---|
| Presentations about various professions | Challenging perceptions – Inter professional relationships |
| Myers Briggs personality test | Challenging perceptions of global, national and local sustainability and impact of midwifery on climate change |

*Table 10.2a* Year Two

| Order of sessions | Cummings and Bennett 6 Cs (2012) focus | Session theme | | Principles -During this session you will: |
|---|---|---|---|---|
| 1 | Communication | 1 | Reflecting on Practice | • Revisit the ground rules set this time last year |
| | | 2 | Documentation | • Use the Southampton Values based model to reflect upon your experiences of practice |
| | | 3 | GDPR | |
| | | 4 | Informed choice | • Explore your own emotional reactions to aspects of practice in relation to both positive and challenging experiences |
| | | | | • Consider the role of effective record keeping in light of realities of practice and NMC requirements |
| | | | | • What is GDPR |
| | | | | • How does GDPR impact on how I keep my documentation? |
| 2 | Compassion and courage | 1 | Learning disabilities | • Review Freddie's story |
| | | 2 | Disability in the workplace | • Advocacy |
| | | | | • Reasonable adjustment |
| | | | | • Inclusivity – what does this mean to me? |
| | | | | • Autism Act |
| 3 | Care and compassion | 1 | Sexuality | • Accepting differences |
| | | 2 | Same sex couples and maternity care | • Acknowledging differences |
| | | | | • Developing openness |
| | | | | • Consideration of the rights of all on maternity care provision |
| | | | | • Advocacy |
| | | | | • Deontology |
| | | | | • Inclusivity |
| 4 | Care commitment | 1 | Case load practice | • Preparation for case-loading linked to autonomous practice module |
| | | 2 | Importance of Multi professional approach in the community | • Health and safety |
| | | | | • Lone working policy |
| | | | | • What does case-loading mean for me |
| | | | | • How would a case-load held model of care fit within my personal life |
| | | | | • Managing competing demands |
| 5 | Care, commitment | 1 | Global perspectives in maternity care | • Sustainable development goals |
| | | | | • World Health organisation |
| | | | | • White ribbon alliance |
| | | | | • Women's health |
| | | | | • Links to Francis report/Kirkup |
| | | | | • World health organisation policy |
| | | | | • Practising midwifery globally |
| | | | | • Cultural competence |

| Order of sessions | Cummings and Bennett 6 Cs (2012) focus | Session theme | | Principles -During this session you will: |
|---|---|---|---|---|
| 6 | Communication, courage | 1 | Stigma | • Tolerance<br>• Acceptance<br>• Awareness<br>• Respect<br>• Advocacy<br>• Human rights |
| 7 | Communication, compassion, courage, care, commitment, competence | 1<br>2 | Communication<br>What happens when multi professional communication fails | • Advance skills<br>• Awareness of self and other<br>• Verbal and non-verbal cues<br>• Scenario based work around failure to communicate. Look at examples |
| 8 | Communication, compassion, courage, care | 1 | Faith, health and culture | • Tolerance/Acceptance<br>• Awareness<br>• Respect<br>• Maternal and fetal/baby death<br>• Conscientious objection and what this means for me<br>• Cultural competence |
| Practice experience 1 | Communication, compassion, courage, care, commitment, competence | Journal club 1 | | • Reviewing evidence based practice<br>• Research into practice<br>• How to apply a critical appraisal to evidence<br>• Focussing on qualitative data<br>• Considering the gaps in knowledge<br>• Developing research understanding and language<br>• How to relate research to client care planning |
| Practice experience 2 | Communication, compassion, courage, care, commitment, competence | Journal club 2 | | • Reviewing evidence based practice<br>• Research into practice<br>• How to apply a critical appraisal to evidence<br>• Focussing on quantitative data<br>• Considering the gaps in knowledge<br>• Developing research understanding and language<br>• How to relate research to client care planning |

*Table 10.2b* Integrating multi professional learning in midwifery using the VBE process

| Case loading – Importance of multi professional working in the community | Attend perinatal mortality meeting to experience multi professional reflection and peer review |
|---|---|
| Communication – To look at the consequences for practice when communication between the professions fails. Case study and mock court room scenario | Be actively involved in daily risk reviews in practice |
| Seek out opportunities to work with other professions during 2nd year | Be proactive in ward round handovers where appropriate |

*Table 10.3a* Year Three

| Order of sessions | Cummings' and Bennett 6 Cs (2012) focus | Session theme | | Principles -During this session you will: |
|---|---|---|---|---|
| 1 | Communication, compassion, courage, care, commitment, competence | 1 | Where am I now in my career trajectory? | • Confidentiality<br>• Sharing practice<br>• Reflection<br>• Developing career planning |
| 2 | Communication, compassion, courage, care, commitment, competence | 1<br>2<br><br>3<br>4<br>5 | Confidence in self<br>Becoming part of the multi-professional team<br>Workforce<br>Courageous leadership<br>Horizontal bullying | • Reflection<br>• Honesty with self<br>• Self-awareness<br>• Support<br>• Development plans<br>• Five dysfunctions of team<br>• Coping with teams when not everyone works as you do<br>• Feeling vulnerable |
| 3 | Communication, care, courage | 1<br>2<br><br>3 | Case study into attitudes<br>Expectations of the public<br>My expectations of others | • What is attitude?<br>• What is an acceptable professional attitude?<br>• Social media sites<br>• Link to mind the gap report<br>• Dealing with frustrations/ feelings wheel<br>• Deflecting behaviours |
| 4 | Communication, compassion, courage, care, commitment, competence | 1 | System failures: case study | • No blame culture/ duty of candour<br>• Openness<br>• Learning<br>• Francis report<br>• Whistleblowing<br>• Escalating concerns |

| Order of sessions | Cummings' and Bennett 6 Cs (2012) focus | Session theme | | Principles -During this session you will: |
|---|---|---|---|---|
| 5 | Communication, compassion, courage, care, commitment, competence | 1<br>2<br>3<br><br>4 | Action learning reflection<br>Anxieties of the future<br>What I am looking forward to most about the future<br>How national policy influences my practice and challenges of current services | • Debriefing<br>• Reflection<br>• Sharing<br>• Moving forward positively<br>• Link to the ten commitments<br>• Fairy tale midwifery |
| 6 | Communication<br>competence, care | 1 | Midwife as educator | • NMC standards for assessing and supervising in practice<br>• Feedback and feed forward<br>• Assessment in practice<br>• Standardisation<br>• Fairness and a just culture<br>• Following processes |
| 7 | Communication, compassion, courage, care, commitment, competence | 1 | Am I the midwife I set out to be? | • Where am I now<br>• Where will I be in 5 years' time<br>• What will my journey look like<br>• How am I building resilience?<br>• Strengthening my capabilities<br>• Strength based approach |
| 8 | Commitment competency | 1 | Preceptorship | • Lifelong learning<br>• Caring/safeguarding for public<br>• Updating knowledge and skills<br>• NMC Rules and standards |
| Practice experience 1 | Communication, compassion, courage, care, commitment, competence | | Journal club 1 | • Implementing my evidence based practice<br>• How my research can inform practice<br>• How to apply a critical appraisal to evidence<br>• How to practice when there are gaps in knowledge<br>• How to relate research to client care planning |
| Practice experience 2 | Communication, compassion, courage, care, commitment, competence | | Journal club 2 | • Implementing my evidence based practice<br>• How my research can inform practice<br>• How to apply a critical appraisal to evidence<br>• How to practice when there are gaps in knowledge<br>• How to relate research to client care planning |

*Table 10.3b* Integrating multi professional learning (MPL) in midwifery using the VBE process

| | |
|---|---|
| • *Confidence in self – becoming an integral member of the multi profession team - Myers Briggs personality test – retest to see how you may have changed throughout your training – strengthening my capabilities – using a strength based approach* | • *Revisit multi professional failings – What is meant by a 'no blame culture' and how does this impact on safety?* |
| • MPL involving service users and student led activity | • Reflect on my personal leadership and coaching others across health care |

## Chapter 4

*Table 10.4* Checklist – see Table 4.1, Chapter 4

| *Themes* | *Supportive information to consider* | *Your comments* | *Completed y/n* |
|---|---|---|---|
| Paperwork and documentation | • Consider what paperwork you need for booking, antenatal appointments, blood tests, referrals etc and ensure that you have these available to you during the visit. If your Trust has electronic forms of documentation, ensure that you have access and if your practice supervisor is required to be present to log you into any online resources.<br>• Think through issues of GDPR (2018). How will you keep records of the interactions you have with women, their families, and other multi-professional groups? If travelling between venues, how will you keep anonymised paper records safely so that if, on the rare occasion, you lost them the details of the woman would not be identifiable?<br>• How will you update any GP and hospital digital records if required?<br>• Does your organisation require you to have all documentation entries countersigned by the responsible practitioner? If so, how will you achieve this? | | |

| Themes | Supportive information to consider | Your comments | Completed y/n |
|---|---|---|---|
| Setting up of case load contract | Best practice ensures completion of a contract between you, your practice supervisor, and the woman.<br><br>● Have you identified and gained agreement to case load with a particular midwife?<br>● How will you work together?<br>● What are the expectations of you and the practice supervisor?<br>● What happens if you are unavailable to attend a planned appointment?<br>● When you have identified your case load, who is going to communicate with the woman to ask if she would like you to case load her?<br>● How will you devise your contract of commitment with the woman?<br>● Does your programme education team/university need to counter sign the contract?<br>● Where will this be stored? | | |
| Yours and your practice supervisor's expectations | ● What do you hope to achieve from this case load experience? Consider a mixture of women for your case load experiences i.e., primiparous, multiparous, VBAC, mental health concerns, safeguarding. Sometimes you are not trying to learn complexity/referrals but 'just' the continuity and being with woman so you may wish for a less complex additional care needs scenario.<br>● Who do you want to case load (in terms of context, learning experience rather than person)?<br>● How many appointments are you expected to attend and how many are reasonable to miss?<br>● How will you undertake a tripartite communication? (you, practice supervisor and woman)<br>● Think through the requirements of the standards for student supervision and assessment (SSSA) (NMC, 2018) and the level you are at in your training. What are the expectations of you at the level of experience you are at, and how do you interpret 'under direct supervision'? You need to be able to work relatively autonomously at some point during the case load so starting from mid-point of your programme is realistic. While it may be a busy time for you, consider how your practice would be different if you did one or two towards the end of training just when you are about to qualify.<br>● How will you demonstrate an ethical understanding of the case load experience and safe professional practice? | | |

| Themes | Supportive information to consider | Your comments | Completed y/n |
|---|---|---|---|
| What are the women's expectations of you? | • Define your professional boundaries before you start so that you are clear prior to discussion of care planning with the woman.<br>• It is strongly recommended that you do not use your personal mobile phone for communications with the client(s). You need to agree with your practice supervisor how you will contact the women on your case load and how they will contact you. It may be that your organisation has a work phone that you can use or a work email. If you use this form of digital communication, remember that this is a contemporary record and professional language must be used. It may be that the women contact you via the Trust's contact number and the Trust contact you.<br>• You need to ensure that the women contact the appropriate departments in the case of a problem as you might not be able to respond to their messages in a timely way<br>• How will you ensure collaborative working/ shared decision-making?<br>• If you make an agreed plan you are expected to be reliable and follow through the activity. | | |
| Planning for the unexpected | • What happens if it goes wrong? Who will you call if you are at a visit on your own and you encounter a problem?<br>• Who do you report back to?<br>• What happens if you are not able to attend at short notice – who do you call i.e., duty manager, midwife, women etc? | | |
| Equipment | • Who in your organisation is responsible for providing students with equipment?<br>• Who is responsible for ensuring the equipment is in working order and restocked?<br>• Some organisations have student case load held bags – if so, where are they stored and are they available when you require them?<br>• Do you have a signing in and out process for borrowing equipment?<br>• Does the practice supervisor or the midwifery team have spare equipment if you want to do a home visit? | | |

| Themes | Supportive information to consider | Your comments | Completed y/n |
|---|---|---|---|
| Risk assessing | • Who has direct accountability and responsibility for the case load and activity?<br>• What responsibility does the Trust and university have towards you and have you completed a risk assessment form for the case load experience? Have you got this countersigned by your practice supervisor and/or midwifery academic assessor (NMC, 2018)<br>• Can you use risk assessment and management strategies to demonstrate adherence to safe practice by ensuring the safety of yourself as a practitioner, your client, and others who you case load? | | |
| Work/life balance | • Have you considered the level of commitment you can provide to the case load at this time in your programme and life circumstances?<br>• Have you considered and agreed travel arrangements and what happens at different time of the day and night? It may be that you use public transport, so consider availability across the day and week<br>• Have you factored in your non-practice obligations and commitments i.e., childcare – school picking up time etc? | | |
| Lone working | • What is the lone working policy of the Trust/ university regarding home visits conducted by a lone student?<br>• Who do you contact to say you are going out to undertake a home visit and what do you do when you have finished the visit?<br>• Do you have a code word or phrase to alert your practice supervisor if you find yourself in an unsafe or emergency situation?<br>• Is it a safe time of day to go to the appointment, e.g., is it in daylight, winter, or summer for the location?<br>• Who will you contact if there are any concerns?<br>• How will you communicate the findings of this visit to the practice supervisor?<br>• Are there any known safeguarding concerns that could comprise your safety?<br>• Are visits and communications outside the agreements permissible? Consider why this would be an issue. | | |

| Themes | Supportive information to consider | Your comments | Completed y/n |
|---|---|---|---|
| Follow up activities | • When referrals need to be made to, for example, consultants, is the practice supervisor in agreement for you to do them and copy them into emails? <br> • If requesting tests and investigations, it is typically the responsibility of the person requesting to follow up on the results. Who will check and action blood results and other tests/investigations? | | |
| Friends and family | • Sometimes you may be approached to case load a friend or member of your family. What are the local guidelines regarding this? <br> • How does this apply to you as a student? <br> • Who do you need to gain permissions from? <br> • How is the role of the PMA used to support this request? | | |

## Case load contract

This contract form can be adapted to meet the requirements of the AEI and NHS Trust that you are assigned to. This resource is based upon one University's suite of case load documents.

Faculty of [*add in your university Faculty name if appropriate*]
School of [*name of school if appropriate*]
University of [*add name of university*]
Student midwife continuity of carer/case load holding documentation 2020/2021

### Confidentiality

Entries made in this document must always ensure confidentiality

[*add image to suit your AEI/NHS Trust*]
Name.................................................................................
Cohort...............................................................................
Academic Tutor/academic assessor................................................
Supervising Midwife................................................................

*What do I need to organise with my supervising midwife?*

Methods of communication with midwife and women.

• Who will approach the women to ask if you can caseload her care and explain what this will entail? Informed consent is vital.
• Your supervising midwife needs to know when you are visiting the woman so she can have it in her diary.

- When you go out to visits in the woman's home you need contact numbers of the midwife and/or the community office. This is because you need to phone to say you have arrived at the visit and then again when you have finished the visit. See lone workers policy.
- You need to discuss with your supervising midwife what will happen in the event of you being unable to attend the visit.
- It is useful to have completed the booking process with at least two of your case load but you can caseload women you have not booked.
- How will you communicate with your supervising midwife the outcome of the visit?
- If the women you are case loading birth in the main unit, how will people know that you are case loading?
- You are expected to visit the women postnatally as needed. You should tailor the postnatal care to the individual, which will not necessarily follow the postnatal guidelines.
- It is important that you have read the contents of this pack and are familiar with the documentation. Sign the risk assessment.
- Your midwife should be doing every other visit with you.
- Please complete reflection sheets in MORA. They will be useful to compare the care you can provide whilst case loading.
- Please complete the client consent form and give the client a copy for their notes

Supervising names and signatures: you are signing to agree that you have read the risk assessment document and are familiar with the local policies to ensure the students work is in accordance with them for their own safety and the safety of the clients.

Supervising Midwife Name............................................

Supervising Midwife Signature....................................

Students Name...........................................................................

Complete the client consent for student continuity of carer/case load held experience per client.

## Chapter 5

### *Consent form*

This consent form can be adapted to meet the requirements of the AEI and NHS Trust that you are assigned to. This form is based upon one University's suite of case load documents.

---

*Place university and/or Trust logo here*
*To whom it may concern*

---

Date _____

Dear _____

Client consent for student continuity of carer/case load held experience.

---

As part of the midwifery education programme, student midwives in their second and third years of training are encouraged to hold a small case load of women. This enables the student to gain important insight and enhances their confidence before qualifying as midwives. The student is closely supported by the practice supervisor. You will see a qualified midwife at least every other appointment and the student will feed back the care that they provide and any concerns that may arise after every appointment. You will also have direct contact numbers for the hospital and the midwife.

It is helpful for students to receive feedback on the care that they are providing and if you feel you can contribute to their leaning you will have the opportunity to fill in a client feedback form.

If you wish to withdraw from the student's case load, please contact the named midwife.

I _____ understand and agree that student midwife _____ will be providing care during my pregnancy, birth and during the postnatal period.

Signatures
Client_____
Student_____
Practice supervisor_____

Contact Numbers
Practice Supervisor_____
Team _____
Community Office_____

Please do not hesitate to contact me, a member of the Midwifery Teaching team at the University of [*name of establishment*], if you wish to discuss any aspect of this student education experience.

Yours sincerely

[Name of responsible midwife teacher or academic assessor]
[Contact details]

*Table 10.5* Risk assessment form adapted from University of Southampton (2020)

| General Health & Safety Risk Assessment Template | | | | | |
|---|---|---|---|---|---|
| **Work activity / task** | 2nd and 3rd year midwifery student's continuity of carer/case load holding | | | | |
| **Assessor(s)** | Name of Module lead | **Responsible Manager** | Name of academic assessor | **Date** | |
| **Faculty/Service** | add | **Academic Unit/Team** | Midwifery | **Location** | Various homes |
| **Brief description of activity / task** | Students will be providing supervised antenatal, intrapartum and postnatal care to clients in their homes as part of the course syllabus by attending client's homes by themselves. | | | | |
| **Additional notes** | *Name Trust* Health and safety Policies on Lone Worker, Infection Control, Sharps Safety, Moving and Handling, Incident Reporting and Clinical Waste should be provided to the student's and read in conjunction with this activity. | | | | |
| **(e.g., references, persons at risk, risk factors, etc) [optional]** | All students will be supervised by a qualified Midwife and students are expected to comply with the NMC professional guidelines. | | | | |
| | Any emergency numbers or working contacts are to be entered into the student's mobile phone for easy access when required. All health and safety requirements set by the Trust in relation to e.g., Covid will be followed. | | | | |
| **Declaration by responsible manager:** I confirm that this is a suitable & sufficient risk assessment for the above work activity/task. | | | | | |
| **Signed** | | **Print name** | Add | **Date** | |
| **Declaration by users:** I confirm that I have read this risk assessment, will implement the controls outlined herein, and will report to the responsible manager any incidents that occur or any shortcomings I find in this assessment. | | | | | |
| **Signed** | | **Print name** | | **Date** | |
| **Signed** | | **Print name** | | **Date** | |
| **Signed** | | **Print name** | | **Date** | |

Health & safety risk assessment: A basic guide
[*add in your AEI policy*]

Table 10.6 Health & safety risk estimation matrix

| Hazards and reasonably foreseeable worst-case consequences | Inherent risk (no controls) from matrix (mark with X) | Controls (measures to reduce risk) | Residual risk (with controls) from matrix (mark with X) |
|---|---|---|---|
| Violence and Aggression toward student from clients or client's partners. | **High** | Trust Lone Worker policy provided to and the student aware of its contents in regard to this activity. | **High** |
| | | NHS has Zero Tolerance controls toward staff and students on honorary employee contracts. | |
| | **Medium** | Risk of domestic violence and higher risk clients (alcohol or drug related) are screened out by qualified Midwives as part of the antenatal assessment of the client prior to case loading to students. | **Medium** |
| | | All students have been trained in conflict resolution as part of the course syllabus which complies with the NHS statutory and mandatory training framework. | |
| | **Low** X | In emergencies students should call (Community Midwives office/supervisor on 00000000000 in the event of escalation of verbal or physical abuse. | **Low** X |
| | | Students record with the community office their destinations and phone in to community office when they arrive and leave a client's premises as part of the safe system of work. | |

| Hazards and reasonably foreseeable worst-case consequences | Inherent risk (no controls) from matrix (mark with X) | Controls (measures to reduce risk) | Residual risk (with controls) from matrix (mark with X) |
|---|---|---|---|
| Biohazards during. | **High** | Trust Safe Sharps Policy provided to students and students aware of the contents as it applies to this activity. | **High** |
| Client Venus blood taking | | UHS Sharps injury reporting policy for needlestick injuries call labour ward on (00000000000 | |
| Client Urine Testing & | | Venus client bloods taken using Vacutainer system to reduce risk. | |
| Baby bloods via heel prick | **Medium** | Disposable Nitrile gloves and aprons to be worn when exposure to blood or urine could occur. | **Medium** |
| | | Baby heel pricks only to be carried out using a safe sharp sprung "lancet". | |
| | **Low** X | Portable sharps containers are carried for the disposal and carriage of used medical sharps. | **Low** X |
| | | Spill kits (swabs and clinical waste bags) available for spillage of bloods or urines and for the carriage of any clinical waste produced in vehicles. | |

| Hazards and reasonably foreseeable worst-case consequences | Inherent risk (no controls) from matrix (mark with X) | | Controls (measures to reduce risk) | Residual risk (with controls) from matrix (mark with X) | |
|---|---|---|---|---|---|
| Biohazard | High | | Clinical waste bags and portable sharps containers are to be always carried. | High | |
| Clinical waste | Medium | | Carriage of waste should be in accordance with Trust Policies and Guidelines and a spill kit containing suitable material to soak up waste and dispose of it for any spills in transit. | Medium | |
| | | | Bloods should be carried in a suitable sealable container that contains a piece of absorbent material if a tube should break. | | |
| | Low | X | | Low | X |
| Hazards and reasonably foreseeable worst case consequences | Inherent risk (no controls) from matrix (mark with X) | | Controls (measures to reduce risk) | Residual risk (with controls) from matrix (mark with X) | |

| Hazards and reasonably foreseeable worst-case consequences | Inherent risk (no controls) from matrix (mark with X) | Controls (measures to reduce risk) | Residual risk (with controls) from matrix (mark with X) |
| --- | --- | --- | --- |
| Musculoskeletal injuries through manual handling of persons and assisting with home deliveries, | High | Students receive patient moving and handling skills training in year one and the skills are practiced and supervised during placements. | High |
|  |  | Students provided with and aware of the contents of Trust manual handling policy as it applies to this activity. |  |
|  | Medium | Students are supervised by qualified Midwife and provide additional support to the Midwife during home births under their direct supervision. | Medium |
|  | Low X |  | Low X |
| Road Traffic Accidents | High | Students own vehicles are insured and carry business class 1 cover for Trust equipment carried. | High |
| Breakdowns - Stranded student) |  | Students must have personal break-down and recovery policies to ensure a suitable response if the vehicle breaks down and they are left isolated in the community. |  |

| Hazards and reasonably foreseeable worst-case consequences | Inherent risk (no controls) from matrix (mark with X) | Controls (measures to reduce risk) | Residual risk (with controls) from matrix (mark with X) |
|---|---|---|---|
| | Medium | All breakdowns/accidents must be reported to the Community Midwives office and the student's supervisor on 00000000000 | Medium |
| | | Students to ensure that they always carry a fully charged mobile phone at the start of the day. And that any emergency numbers, community Midwives office and supervisors' numbers are entered into the mobile phone for expediency of access. | |
| | Low    X | | Low    X |
| Covid related restrictions and safe practice | High | All students are required to follow the latest Trust guidance related to community visits, case loading and Covid | High |
| | Medium | | Medium    x |
| | Low | | Low |

| Hazards and reasonably foreseeable worst-case consequences | Inherent risk (no controls) from matrix (mark with X) | Controls (measures to reduce risk) | Residual risk (with controls) from matrix (mark with X) |
|---|---|---|---|
| | High | | High |

Note: **High risk** – requires controls to reduce risk before activity / task can commence (or continue).
Note: **Medium risk** – requires controls to reduce risk as much and as soon as is reasonably practicable.
Note: **Low risk** – all risk should be reduced to this tolerable level, so far as is reasonably practicable.

# Chapter 6

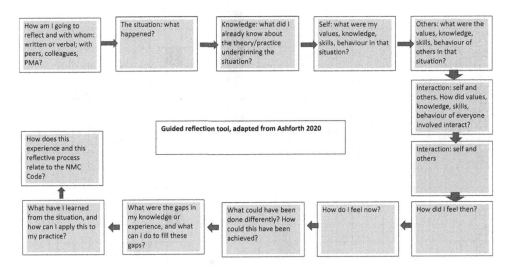

*Figure 10.1* Guided reflection tool, adapted from Ashforth 2020

# Chapter 7

*Table 10.7* SMARTER objectives (NHS England, 2020)

| Specific | Measur-able | Achievable | Realistic/ relevant | Timed | Evaluate | Readjust |
|---|---|---|---|---|---|---|
| What is the action/objective to be achieved? | How will you know you have met the objective? | Is this possible to achieve? | Is this relevant to your role? | How long will this take? | Did it go to plan? | Do you need to read just the original actions to achieve? |

# Chapter 8

| WEEK | 1 | 2 | 3 | 4 | 5 | 6 | 7 | 8 | 9 | 10 | 11 | 12 | 13 | 14 | 15 | 16 | 17 | 18 | 19 | 20 | 21 | 22 | 23 | 24 | 25 | 26 | 27 | 28 | 29 | 30 |
|------|---|---|---|---|---|---|---|---|---|----|----|----|----|----|----|----|----|----|----|----|----|----|----|----|----|----|----|----|----|----|
| **TASK** | | | | | | | | | | | | | | | | | | | | | | | | | | | | | | |
| Proposal | ■ | ■ | | | | | | | | | | | | | | | | | | | | | | | | | | | | |
| Submission | | | ■ | | | | | | | | | | | | | | | | | | | | | | | | | | | |
| Feedback from peer review | | | | | ■ | | | | | | | | | | | | | | | | | | | | | | | | | |
| Respond to feedback | | | | | | ■ | ■ | | | | | | | | | | | | | | | | | | | | | | | |
| Ethics process and paperwork | | | ■ | ■ | | | ■ | | | | | | | | | | | | | | | | | | | | | | | |
| Submission | | | | | | | | ■ | | | | | | | | | | | | | | | | | | | | | | |
| Sampling | | | | | | | | | | | ■ | ■ | ■ | | ■ | ■ | | | | | | | | | | | | | | |
| Data collection | | | | | | | | | | | | | | ■ | | ■ | ■ | | | | | | | | | | | | | |
| Data analysis | | | | | | | | | | | | | | | | | | | | | | | | | | | | | | |
| Write up | | | | | | | | | ■ | ■ | | | | | | ■ | | | | | ■ | | | ■ | ■ | ■ | | | | |
| Submission | | | | | | | | | | | | | | | | | | | | | ■ | ■ | | | | | | ■ | ■ | |
| Log book | | ■ | ■ | | | | | | | | | | ■ | ■ | | | | | | ■ | ■ | | | | | | | | | |
| Supervision | ■ | | | | | | | ■ | | | | | | | | | ■ | | | | | | | | | ■ | | | | |
| Placement | | | | | | ■ | ■ | ■ | ■ | ■ | ■ | ■ | ■ | ■ | ■ | | | | | | | | | | | | | | | |
| Module | | | | | | | | | | | | | | | | | ■ | ■ | ■ | ■ | ■ | ■ | ■ | | | | | | | |
| Module essay writing | | | | | | | | | | | | | | | | | | | | | | | ■ | ■ | | | | | | |
| Module essay submission | | | | | | | | | | | | | | | | | | | | | | | | | ■ | | | | | |

*Figure 10.2* GANTT chart – worked example

*Table 10.8* GANTT chart – blank example for you to modify

| WEEK<br>*(date, month or week number)*<br><br>TASK | | | | *Add more col-umns as required* |
|---|---|---|---|---|
| | | | | |
| Proposal | | | | |
| Submission | | | | |
| Feedback from peer review | | | | |
| Respond to feedback | | | | |
| Ethics process and paperwork | | | | |
| Submission | | | | |
| Sampling | | | | |
| Data collection | | | | |
| Data analysis | | | | |
| Write up | | | | |
| Submission | | | | |
| Log book | | | | |
| Supervision | | | | |
| Placement | | | | |
| Module | | | | |
| Module essay writing | | | | |
| Module essay submission | | | | |
| | | | | |
| *Add more rows as required* | | | | |

*Table 10.9* Sample contents page for portfolio of work

| Section/heading | Notes | Completed |
| --- | --- | --- |
| Title page | | |
| Initial reflection on practice: recognising bias and a priori knowledge | | |
| Introduction: rationale for choice of project area; definition of terms used, including abbreviations; local and national guidelines pertaining to the project area | | |
| Literature search with inclusion and exclusion criteria, and search terms, search results, initial critique of the literature to identify articles for review | | |
| Critical review of the literature | | |
| Methodology used, and rationale for doing so | | |
| Sampling, including inclusion/exclusion criteria | | |
| Identifying and recruiting eligible participants, including flow chart for use in practice | | |
| Project information pack: letter of invitation to participate, participant information sheet, contact details sheet | | |
| Data collection, including example of data collection tool (eg interview guide, questionnaire, survey) | | |
| Data analysis: data (e.g. interview transcripts, questionnaire results), and data analysis tool, such as thematic framework. Coding, data summary and organisation of themes. Linking the themes to the literature) | | |
| Discussion and implications for practice | | |
| Ethics and data management: good clinical practice certificate, Health Research Authority decision tree, letter of support/permission from the Trust, peer review, University ethics approval | | |
| Project protocol | | |
| Record of supervision | | |
| Final reflection | | |
| Bibliography | | |
| Final written piece for submission | | |

*Table 10.10* Sample headings page for protocol

| Section/sub-heading | Notes | Completed |
|---|---|---|
| Background, synopsis of literature | | |
| Rationale for project | | |
| Aim and objectives | | |
| Methodology | | |
| Setting of project | | |
| Study population | | |
| Recruitment | | |
| Data collection | | |
| Data analysis | | |
| Dissemination of findings | | |
| Ethics and data management | | |
| Project finance | | |
| Reference list | | |
| Appendix A: NHS Health Research Authority decision tree | | |
| Appendix B: Reflection on practice | | |
| Appendix C: Letter of invitation to participate | | |
| Appendix D: Participant information sheet | | |
| Appendix E: Contact details sheet | | |
| Appendix F: Lone working policy and risk-assessment | | |
| Appendix G: Consent form | | |
| Appendix H: Data collection tool | | |
| Appendix I: Project plan and GANTT chart | | |

### Service evaluation -v- audit -v- research -v- quality improvement project

It is often challenging to distinguish between service evaluation, audit, quality improvement projects and research. This table based on Twycross and Shorten (2014) and Tasker (2013) aims to show you the differences. The final column is for you to make comments to see which study type best meets the question that you are seeking the answer to.

*Table 10.11* Service evaluation -v- audit -v- research -v- quality improvement project

| Study type | Characteristics | Comments |
| --- | --- | --- |
| Service evaluation – seeks to assess how well a service is achieving its intended aims. | Aim to judge the quality of the current service <br>     Initiated by service providers <br>     Does not involve a new treatment <br>     No randomisation <br>     Does not allocate patients to treatment groups | |
| Audit – systematically looks at the procedures used for diagnosis, care, and treatment, examining how associated resources are used and investigating the effect care has on the outcome and quality of life for the patient (DH, 2003) | Aim to measure clinical practice against a standard <br>     Initiated by service providers <br>     Does not involve a new treatment <br>     No randomisation <br>     Does not allocate patients to treatment groups | |
| Quality improvement project – the process by which better patient experience and outcomes are "achieved through changing provider behaviour and organisation through using a systematic change method and strategies (Tasker, 2013) | Aim to improve patient care by making small incremental changes and measurements which maybe done weekly to test the impact of the changes. | |
| Research – involves the attempt to extend the available knowledge by means of systematically defensible process of enquiry (Clamp et al, 2004) | Aim to generate new knowledge/add to the body of knowledge <br>     Initiated by researchers <br>     Sometimes involves a new treatment <br>     Sometimes have randomisation <br>     Sometimes allocates patients to treatment groups | |

# Chapter 9

*Table 10.12* One-, three- and five-year plan

| Plan time scales | Where do I see myself in 1/ 3/5 years' time? List aspirations/activities | Education and development needs analysis. List resources required to achieve your ambition. | Timescale? |
|---|---|---|---|
| 1 year | e.g., Consolidate pre-registration preparation<br>e.g., Complete preceptorship programme | | |
| 3 years | | | |
| 5 years | | | |

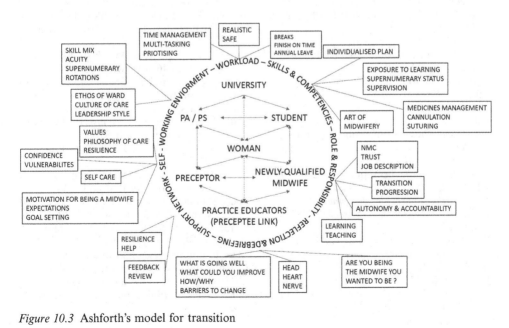

*Figure 10.3* Ashforth's model for transition

# Index

Page numbers in *italics* refer to figures. Page numbers in **bold** refer to tables.

Printed in the United States
by Baker & Taylor Publisher Services